C000099402

PAIN-FREE
HORSE RIDING

An Illustrated Guide to Prevention, Self-Care,
and Injury Management for Riders of All Abilities

Nikki Robinson

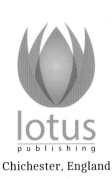

lotus
publishing

Chichester, England

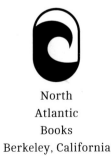

North
Atlantic
Books

Berkeley, California

First published in 2018
Lotus Publishing
Apple Tree Cottage, Inlands Road, Nutbourne, Chichester, PO18 8RJ, and
North Atlantic Books
Berkeley, California

Illustrations Gabrielle Vickery Illustration
Photographs Maria T. Michael of Detheo Photography, unless otherwise indicated
Text Design Medlar Publishing Solutions Pvt Ltd., India
Cover Design Chris Fulcher
Printed and Bound in India by Replika Press

Pain-Free Horse Riding: An Illustrated Guide to Prevention, Self-Care, and Injury Management for Riders of All Abilities is sponsored and published by the Society for the Study of Native Arts and Sciences (dba North Atlantic Books), an educational nonprofit based in Berkeley, California, that collaborates with partners to develop cross-cultural perspectives, nurture holistic views of art, science, the humanities, and healing, and seed personal and global transformation by publishing work on the relationship of body, spirit, and nature.

North Atlantic Books' publications are available through most bookstores. For further information, visit our website at www.northatlanticbooks.com or call 800-733-3000.

British Library Cataloguing-in-Publication Data
A CIP record for this book is available from the British Library
ISBN 978 1 905367 92 4 (Lotus Publishing)
ISBN 978 1 623173 67 8 (North Atlantic Books)

Library of Congress Cataloging-in-Publication Data
Names: Robinson, Nikki, 1970- author.
Title: Pain-free horse riding : an illustrated guide to prevention,
    self-care, and injury management for riders of all abilities / Nikki
    Robinson; foreword by John Barnes, PT.
Description: North Atlantic Books edition. | Berkeley, California : North
    Atlantic Books, 2019. | First published in 2018 by Lotus Publishing Apple
    Tree Cottage. | Includes bibliographical references and index.
Identifiers: LCCN 2018033811 (print) | LCCN 2018034703 (ebook) | ISBN
    9781623173685 (E-book) | ISBN 9781623173678 (trade paper)
Subjects: LCSH: Horsemanship--Physiological aspects. | Equestrian
    accidents--Prevention.
Classification: LCC RC1220.H67 (ebook) | LCC RC1220.H67 R63 2019 (print) |
    DDC 615.8/51581--dc23
LC record available at https://lccn.loc.gov/2018033811

Contents

Important note

Acknowledgments

Huge thanks and appreciation to my long-suffering family—Pete, Freddy, Joey, and Katie—who had to put up with me focusing on nothing but writing this book for five months.

Also, thanks to the amazing team at Holisticare and my lovely patients for their encouragement and making me believe that I was capable of putting my passion into words.

Thank you to Mel at Attridges Equestrian Centre for providing the perfect location for our photo shoot. Also, huge appreciation to Mel and all the staff and liveries at Attridges for their help, advice and support.

Maria the photographer and Gabrielle the illustrator: you are very talented and it was a pleasure to work with both of you. I learnt a lot and I think that we made a great team.

I really appreciate the lovely words written by John F. Barnes in the Foreword and by Sarah, Duchess of York, and Laura Renwick in their quotes for this book.

Jamie and Arlyse, Jess and Hannah, and Lara: thank you for your generosity in allowing me to use your images.

Thank you to Sally, Katie, and Tracy for patiently reading through what I had written and giving great feedback, and to my friends and networking buddies for their support and introductions.

This book wouldn't be the same without the words from my patients about their experiences, or the models Katie, Brooke, Louise, and Dan. Thank you all so much for your generosity and for being part of this book.

Jon at Lotus Publishing and Emily at North Atlantic Books: thank you for your help and for trusting me to deliver my book in the right way.

Foreword

I have had the honor and opportunity of knowing Nikki Robinson for a number of years through my Myofascial Release seminars. She is a highly intelligent, excellent therapist, who has combined her love of horses with her expertise in Myofascial Release.

I have had a love of animals for my whole life. I have been treating equine athletes for decades now, with great success. I am a physical therapist that has been treating humans, horses and a variety of animals from all over the world that have gotten into serious trouble. When other forms of traditional therapy unfortunately did not help them, Myofascial Release did. Myofascial Release is the missing link in health care for both humans and animals!

I was an athlete when I was younger and I fell with 300 pounds in a weight lifting contest which ruptured a disc in my lower back area. I tried every form of therapy including surgery to get better, nothing worked. There was a day when I realized that there's nobody going to help me, but me. Nobody wanted to get better more than I, I started to treat myself on my living room floor. Over time, I started to make a remarkable recovery. I then utilized these principles, which are totally different than other forms of traditional therapy, on my patients.

Science is verifying the principles of Myofascial Release that I have been teaching now for over 40 years. Fascia is an incredibly powerful connective tissue that connects and intersperses with every muscle, bone, nerve, organ, cell in our body. When restricted, fascial restrictions can generate tensile forces of up to approximately 2,000 pounds per square inch of pressure. Crushing pressure! The important point here also is that fascial restrictions do not show up in any of the standard testing that is currently being offered for humans or animals; x-rays, CAT scans, blood work, etc. Therefore, fascial restrictions have been misdiagnosed for eons. A highly trained therapist, such as Nikki, can feel where the restrictions lie in a particular individual. Fascial restrictions can lead to pain, restriction of motion, and a multitude of symptoms.

I got a call one day from a friend that had race horses. He had just purchased a horse that had great confirmation and amazing potential, but every time they would run the horse he would go lame within a hundred yards. I went to the stable with my friend and started to apply my Myofascial Release principles. In three treatments, this beautiful horse was running a mile without veering off his center, was totally different in his gait, fluidity of motion and increased power. With 3 months of further training he went on to win, and shatter, the record for three year olds at Belmont Stakes Park which is the famous racetrack outside of New York City. This horse was purchased for $19,000 and after I treated him, six months later, he had won over $600,000.

Myofascial Release principles are safe, highly effective for everybody. I cannot more strongly recommend that you follow Nikki's advice. She has an amazing perspective with how to treat horseback riders.

John F. Barnes PT

Introduction

◼ IS THIS YOU?

If you relate to any of these statements, then this book could help you to find the answers:

- ☐ I am in constant pain or discomfort.
- ☐ My sleep is often disturbed by pain.
- ☐ I can't do the activities I want to because of my pain.
- ☐ I need daily medication to control my pain.
- ☐ I can't stand or walk for very long.

- ☐ I can't ride as much as I would like to because of my symptoms.
- ☐ I am always being told to correct my posture when I ride.
- ☐ I have had several falls from horses over the years.
- ☐ I can only look after my horse if I take painkillers.
- ☐ I limit what I do when riding now so that my symptoms don't flare up.

- ☐ I have to plan my days around my body.
- ☐ I usually manage my symptoms but sometimes a small event can make everything flare up.
- ☐ If I have a good day I tend to overdo it, because I have to make the most of it.
- ☐ I can't keep up with friends of the same age as me.
- ☐ I have to take my own pillow if I go away.

- ☐ My body stiffens up over night.
- ☐ I feel as though I am tied up in knots.
- ☐ Stretching helps, but I can't get far enough.
- ☐ I find it difficult to stand straight when I get up from sitting.
- ☐ It is very difficult for me to relax.

- ☐ I get very anxious and frustrated about my symptoms.
- ☐ I find myself waiting for my pain to return.
- ☐ I have been told it's all in my head.
- ☐ There is no point in having more treatment as I have tried everything.
- ☐ I have to ignore my body to get through the day.

- ☐ I have been told that my pelvis is out of alignment.
- ☐ I was given orthotics but they didn't make any difference.
- ☐ My bite is out of line.
- ☐ I feel off balance.
- ☐ One of my legs feels longer than the other.

- ☐ I have tried lots of different treatments.
- ☐ I have been told that I can't be helped.
- ☐ My symptoms move around and change.
- ☐ My symptoms don't all fit into one diagnosis.
- ☐ My body is hypersensitive.

In a recent survey of horse riders undertaken by the author, one hundred percent of respondents stated that they are living with pain. There are so many people riding and working with horses, and all are very likely to have pain that affects their riding and activities at some point. If you are one of those, please use this book to help you to identify what you can do to help yourself.

■ HOW TO USE THIS BOOK

It has been said to me that "riders don't read books"!

So, this book is perfect for horse people of all abilities and of any age who simply don't have the time or inclination to read a book. It is easy to pick up and browse, giving simple, practical, and commonsense tips on how to reduce your pain. If you have a specific problem that you need help with, you can just turn straight to that section to find what you are looking for. You won't have to read it cover to cover, and there are plenty of photographs and illustrations to explain each point.

However, if you do enjoy reading a book from start to finish, there is a lot of information and explanation of how your body works and why you feel what you feel, relating to the latest research. This leads on to practical advice that is applicable to your riding and work on the yard. If you would like to find out more details about the facts, there are references throughout the book for you to look up.

In this way, even if you are a rider who thinks that it is OK to live with pain, you can gain knowledge and understanding of your body. And the sooner you act on this knowledge, the longer you will be able to continue riding and caring for your horse.

■ WHY I WROTE THIS BOOK

Physiotherapy (physical therapy)

I decided that I wanted to be a physiotherapist (physical therapist) when I spoke to one at a school careers evening, aged thirteen. Luckily, this teenage choice led me to a profession that has taken me around the world, fits around my family commitments, and fulfills me every day.

In 1993, I graduated from the Queen Elizabeth School of Physiotherapy in Birmingham in the UK, after three years of training. My first job was at the Luton and Dunstable Hospital in Bedfordshire, where I spent two years rotating through the specialties, gaining a broad base of knowledge and experience.

From the beginning, working in a hospital outpatients' department didn't feel that it suited me. I didn't like only being allowed to treat the part of my patient's body that the doctor wrote on the referral letter. However, I loved working on the wards, where I was free to treat my patients in my own way, especially in trauma and orthopedics.

After eighteen months I was given a fantastic opportunity: I swapped jobs with an Australian physiotherapist and went to live and work in Victoria for three months. That led to various locum positions in Melbourne, with a fair bit of traveling along the way!

On my return to the UK, following a honeymoon backpacking through India and Nepal, I did some more locum jobs. Then I settled at the Thurrock Community Trust in Essex, as a superintendent physiotherapist. This gave me wonderful experience in working within a great multidisciplinary team and managing community therapists.

In 2001 I left to look after my baby twin boys, who were joined by a baby sister three years later. As you can imagine, this took up all my time and energy for a few years! But when my daughter started playgroup in 2006, I decided to set up my own physiotherapy practice. That was when I remembered that I didn't enjoy outpatients.

So I started researching some courses that I could take to update my skills, and that is how I came across Myofascial Release.

Myofascial release

After the first five minutes of my first Myofascial Release course, I felt that I had come home. It sounds corny, I know, but suddenly all my concerns about working with outpatients fell away.

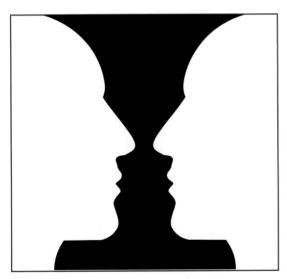

Observing the same thing from a different perspective.

This is the illustration that had an immediate impact on me. In all those years of treating people, I had been looking at the wrong picture! By learning how to observe and feel in the correct way, I felt that I was now able to work with my patients to change their symptoms.

I specialized in Myofascial Release straight away, and it has taken me on an amazing personal and professional journey that still continues today.

My initial Myofascial Release courses were in the UK, and I then trained in America with John Barnes, the physiotherapist who developed the technique. But, of course, learning is a continuous process and I still travel to the US to train with him whenever I can.

Since specializing in Myofascial Release, I have worked with thousands of patients who have had a huge variety of symptoms and conditions. The scope of this treatment continues to amaze and impress me.

Horses

I learnt to ride as a child but didn't have the opportunity to spend a lot of time with horses, although I was always drawn to them whenever it was possible.

It was when my daughter started to have weekly lessons that I felt an increasing need to ride again, but it took over a year for me to build up the courage to speak to the instructor and have a go. That first lesson felt like it was my first time ever on a horse! My muscle memory and balance seemed to have completely deserted me, but I loved it.

Fast-forward a few years of me riding occasionally and my daughter begging me almost constantly to have her own horse, and I finally realized that actually I would like to own one too. So we looked for a horse that would be suitable for both of us to share, and in February 2017 we found Clover. She is a 16.2 hh Irish draft X, and she has changed our lives. Our learning curve (particularly mine) has been huge, and I now can't imagine life without a horse in it.

Combining my two passions

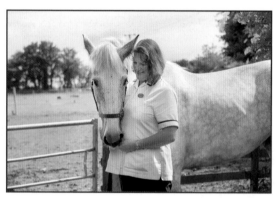

Nikki with Clover.

In my physiotherapy practice many of my patients are or have been horse riders. When taking their medical history, I have learnt to ask, "And how about falls?" if they even mention horses or riding. This is because, unless they have been taken to hospital in the back of an ambulance, a fall from a horse doesn't seem to be a memory of any significance to them.

I have met so many ex-riders who would have loved to continue, but simply couldn't as their bodies are so broken. The wistful look in their eyes when they tell me about horses they have owned and how they used to love riding was one of my motivators for writing this book.

Every groom or yard worker that I have spoken to is living with pain of some sort, but they all turn up for work every day in all weathers. After their working day is finished, many of them then have to start mucking out and caring for their own horse. If they are lucky and they are not in too much pain, there might also be time for a ride.

The reality is that every impact affects your whole body and has the potential to cause problems in the future if it is not treated. Horse riders are not immune to this impact, and yet it has become normal to get up and carry on after a fall as though nothing has happened. In fact, if there are any witnesses they will usually encourage the fallen rider to get back in the saddle as soon as possible. This has led to a culture of not only accepting pain, but of being thought of as showing weakness if you take time out or accept treatment for anything less than a broken bone.

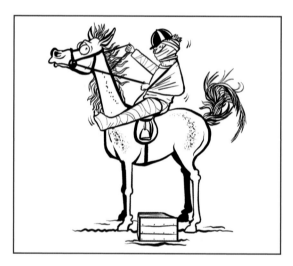

The more time that I spent on the yard, working with and speaking to other horse lovers, the more I realized that there is no need to accept this. That is why I have written this book, and I sincerely hope that reading it will allow you to find some answers and solutions so that you don't have to live with pain.

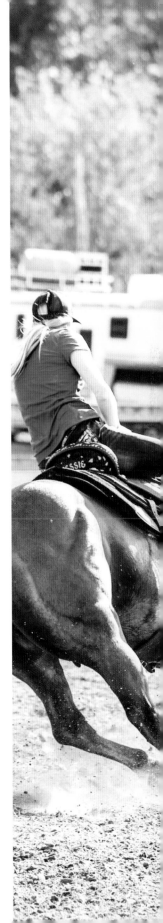

CHAPTER 1

The Rider's Posture

■ THE BENEFITS OF RIDING

The most recent British Equestrian Trade Association (BETA) National Equestrian Survey in 2015 indicated that 2.7 million people in the UK ride, with ninety-six percent riding for pleasure.[1] Of the ex-riders, thirty-four percent would like to return to riding in the future. The estimated British horse population, including both private and professional ownership, is 944,000.

According to the Equestrian Channel's US horse-industry statistics, there are 9.2 million horses in the United States, with 4.6 million people involved in the horse industry in some way.[2]

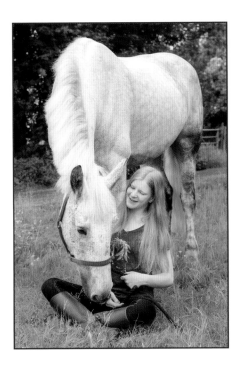

A study undertaken by the University of Brighton on behalf of the British Horse Society found that there are physical, psychological, and well-being benefits of horse riding.[3] The researchers found that riding and activities such as mucking out could be classed as "moderate-intensity exercise," and that horse riding stimulates positive feelings, leading to a sense of well-being. Riding and caring for your horse are a complete workout both physically and mentally.

A Japanese study found that children who rode horses demonstrated an improved ability to recognize appropriate responses (go and no-go reactions) to situations, and a higher level of appropriate self-control.[4] This was thought to be caused by the effect of the horse's vibrations in the different paces on the nervous system. The researchers also noticed a reduction in children's stress levels with some horses.

All riders have their own story about how and why they began their relationship with horses. But whether or not you ride regularly, you can still benefit from contact with these amazing creatures. I sincerely hope that you are able to stay pain free so that you can enjoy your horse for as long as possible.

■ THE IDEAL POSTURE

The classical riding seat, which can mostly be seen in dressage, was developed in the late nineteenth and early twentieth centuries. In this position, the rider is balanced and upright, with equal weight through both sides of the rider's pelvis into the feet. The spine position is neutral with the shoulders relaxed and level. It should be possible to drop a theoretical plumb line down from the ear to the shoulder, through the elbow and hip, and into the ankle bone.

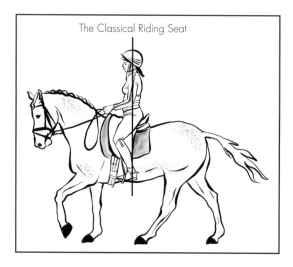

By starting with a good posture it is much easier to feel your horse and to be able to go through the paces without putting strain on your own or your horse's body. Ideally, the rider should be toned and relaxed at the same time. This means that you are alert enough to respond to your horse and to ask for the horse to respond to you, but relaxed enough to soften and feel what your horse is doing under you without putting undue pressure on it.

Professional dressage riders demonstrate the most classical seat in modern riding, moving as one with their horses and able to apply the aids so subtly that it appears to the untrained eye that they are doing nothing. Of course, we know that this is only attained at the very highest level, but it is something that a lot of riders aspire to.

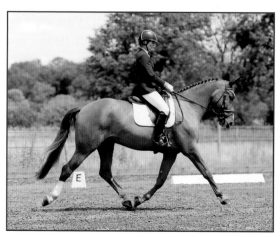

Photograph courtesy of John Tyrrell.

From the time that we start to learn to ride, maybe as children, we are told to sit straight, with our elbows in, toes pointing forward, heels down, etc. But even if we start riding at a young age, it is actually very difficult to maintain this posture. The reason for this has not so much to do with strength or lack of talent, and a lot to do with what you and your body have been through in your life up to that point, including how you were born.

So, your ideal or optimum posture is likely to be different from other people's, as only your body has had your experiences. Of course I am not saying that we shouldn't aspire to riding with as good a posture as possible, but your route to that posture will be individual to you.

■ THE REALITY

The reality is that we are not made up of bones stacked up one on top of the other. Your skeletal system is actually held within your soft tissue, and your bones have to constantly adapt to the pulls and pushes of the rest of your body. By trying to achieve that perfect plumb-line posture, many riders are putting more strain on their bodies, and also on their horses, because they try to force it. So while this posture may be possible to achieve with the correct training for you and your horse and by receiving treatment as you both need it, that is not the reality for most riders.

Some of my patients with the worst posture and the tightest muscles are those who were told as children to stand up straight and keep their shoulders back. Some were even made to walk around with a stick across the back of their shoulders! This has resulted in a spine that is ramrod straight and shoulders held in extreme tension. While the body is being held in this way, their whole system is put under so much tension that they are unable to adapt to any stresses that come along.

Did you know that most people are walking around with a wonky pelvis?

Your pelvis is made up of two bones, and the muscles attaching to those bones are the strongest in the body: those in your legs, back, and stomach.

Throughout your life, injuries and strains to those muscles cause them to tighten up. If they tighten asymmetrically they exert a rotational force on the bones of your pelvis, which causes those bones to gradually creep out of position. Because it happens slowly, the brain adapts to it, so most people are unaware that their pelvis is out of alignment. It can make you feel that you are off balance, and often people are told that one leg is longer than the other. It can also throw your shoulders out of position.

- Are your stirrup leathers different lengths?
- Does your saddle always twist to the same side?
- Do you find it much harder to canter on one rein?

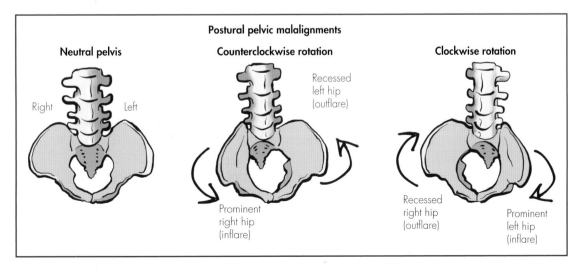

Postural pelvic malalignments

Neutral pelvis

Right　　Left

Counterclockwise rotation

Recessed left hip (outflare)

Prominent right hip (inflare)

Clockwise rotation

Recessed right hip (outflare)

Prominent left hip (inflare)

A rotated pelvis makes it very hard to maintain the classical riding position. The resulting muscle tightness means that some muscle groups will be working harder than they should and might be very hard to relax, and others may appear to be weak and difficult to use properly.

Apart from your pelvis, there are other areas where bony abnormalities may be pulling you out of that plumb-line position:

* Scoliosis is a curve in your spine that can simply be a result of pelvic rotation, but may also be a more serious problem from your childhood.
* Fractures to any bone leave scarring and possibly altered alignment.
* Arthritic changes alter the balance of a joint.

Any of these changes will cause the surrounding muscles to have to change their alignment too, with a knock-on effect on other bones and joints.

■ HOW YOUR POSTURE AFFECTS YOUR RIDING

Your skeleton only has the structure that it has because of the soft tissue holding the bones in their relative positions—without it you would simply be a pile of bones. So, if your muscles are tight your whole skeleton will be pulled out of position. This makes it extremely difficult to achieve a toned and balanced posture. Muscles can appear weak if they are tight or twisted. Often, riding instructors will repeatedly tell their pupils to pull their shoulders back, put their heels down, and sit up straight. The reason this is so difficult to maintain is that tension within your body is pulling you into different positions.

Muscles in your body tend to work in pairs, often front to back; for example, your biceps

and triceps muscles in your upper arm. In order for one muscle to work effectively (the agonist), its opposite muscle must be able to relax (the antagonist).

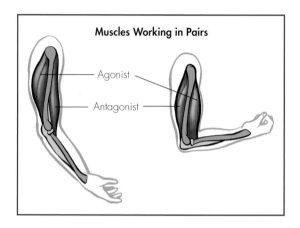

Muscles Working in Pairs

Agonist

Antagonist

Therefore, if you have tension that you can't let go of, the opposite muscle group will not be able to work correctly. This will have a big impact on your riding when you are trying to keep your hands soft and your seat light. Another implication of your alignment is the way that weight is transferred down your body as you are riding. If you are tense and in the wrong position, it will be difficult to feel what your horse is doing under you. The more out of alignment you are, the harder it is to stay balanced, meaning that you are more likely to fall off.

Of course, your horse's muscles also work in this way, with one set of muscles needing to let go to allow the opposing muscles to work effectively. So imagine how much more difficult it must be for your horse to do this, if your agonist/antagonist balance is out in multiple muscle groups.

■ HOW YOUR POSTURE AFFECTS YOUR HORSE

I recently met a rider who told me that she'd had a very bad fall, fracturing her pelvis. After a long period of rehabilitation, she had tried to ride her horse again, but each time it was stirring up her pain so she had to take another break from riding. She then asked a professional trainer to come once a week to school her horse. After the first time, he told her that there had to be a major problem with her horse's back, as he was in pain after riding him. They couldn't find any pain or lameness in the horse, but the trainer kept feeling that his body was being thrown out by the horse. That was when this lady realized that it must have been her body that the horse was compensating for. They are now working on correcting the horse's posture and the owner is going to come and have her pelvis balanced before she rides again.

Your center of gravity has a direct affect on your horse's center of gravity. Remember that your horse should be balanced without a rider, so even a perfectly aligned rider will affect the horse.

Twists in your body mean that your horse has to compensate continually while being ridden. Even if the horse has its back treated, the problem will recur if the rider isn't treated too. That is why riders who own more than one horse will often notice similar problems in all their horses.

All horses have a tendency to bend more easily to one direction than the other, causing one side to be more rounded and the other more hollow. Riders tend to get pushed over to the hollow side, which will cause the horse to have to compensate and alter its center of gravity.

The trouble is that most riders also have an easier side that they tend to lean toward. So your horse has to adapt to your off-center center of gravity, as well having to adapt to the effect that its own posture is having on your seat. Then even walking in a straight line becomes an exercise in balance and coordination for your horse. It is easy to

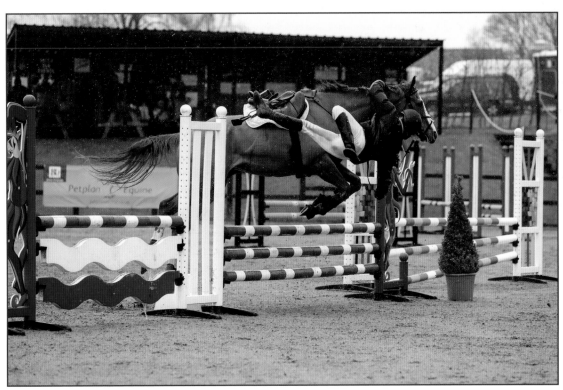

Photograph courtesy of Spencer Moret.

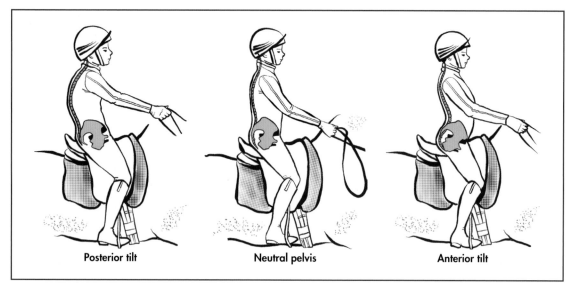

| Posterior tilt | Neutral pelvis | Anterior tilt |

The effect of pelvic rotation when riding.

understand why things can go wrong so quickly when we ask our horses to push themselves.

Saddles will also change shape according to the stresses put on them. This means that they will need to be checked after both the horse and rider have been treated. The male and female pelvises are different shapes, and male and female riders sit very differently in their saddles.

According to Australian saddler Peter Horobin, ninety percent of riders are women but saddles are mostly made for the male anatomy.[5] This was first recognized by Dr. Deb Bennett in 1989.[6] She talked about the Native American tribes that built different types of saddles for men and women, which were adapted for their different uses but also to reflect their differing anatomy. She suggested that these differences mean that men and women have different issues when learning to ride, and when competing in certain disciplines such as dressage and eventing.

The female pelvis is larger and wider, with a circular pelvic inlet (opening at the base of the pelvis), making the hip sockets further apart. A woman's sacrum (the fused vertebrae at the base of the spine) is also tilted further back than a man's. These features are to allow for ease of childbirth.

When women sit in a saddle, they naturally have their weight toward the front of their pelvis, which extends or hollows their lower back. When this is exaggerated, it increases tension in the upper back and causes the chin to stick out.

The male pelvis is longer and narrower, with a heart-shaped pelvic inlet and straighter sacrum. The male rider's hip sockets are oriented more to the front than the female rider's, and he is more likely to have a slouched posture in the saddle when he relaxes his lower back.

So, if you share a horse with someone of the opposite sex, you are likely to need a separate saddle for each of you. This is not only important for the comfort and health of the riders, but also for their horse. If the weight of the rider is wrongly distributed, it will affect the horse's body even if the fit of the saddle is good.

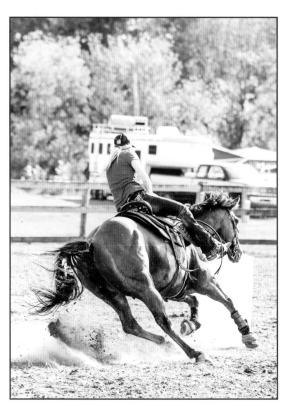

Photograph courtesy of @kyliesheaforphotog via Twenty20.

You should also bear in mind that riders of the same sex will have varying needs when it comes to saddle size and fit. This can be catered for by a good saddle fitter. For example, my daughter and I share our mare and we are a very different size and shape to each other. I need to add a gel pad under the saddle when I am riding to alter the weight distribution and balance the saddle correctly.

Different types of riding mean that both horses and riders need to train for the specific requirements of each discipline or activity. Some breeds of horse are naturally suited to a particular style of riding, and it is the same for the riders. But even they will have to train their bodies to adapt to how they need to sit and move during their chosen activity in order to attain any level of achievement.

■ REFERENCES

1. British Equestrian Trade Association (BETA). "National Equestrian Survey 2015 Shows Increased Consumer Spending." BETA. Last modified 2015, accessed 16 June 2018. http://www.beta-uk.org/pages/news-amp-events/news/national-equestrian-survey-2015-shows-increased-consumer-spending.php.

2. Equestrian Channel. "US Horse Industry Statistics." Equestrian Channel. N.d., accessed 16 June 2018. http://www.theequestrianchannel.com/id3.html.

3. British Horse Society. "The Health Benefits of Horse Riding in the UK." British Horse Society. Last modified 2011, accessed 16 June 2018. http://www.bhs.org.uk/enjoy-riding/health-benefits.

4. N. Ohtani, K. Kitagawa, K. Mikami, K. Kitawaki, J. Akiyama, M. Fuchikami, H. Uchiyama, and M. Ohta. "Horseback Riding Improves the Ability to Cause the Appropriate Action (Go Reaction) and the Appropriate Self-Control (No-Go Reaction) in Children." *Frontiers in Public Health* (6 February 2017). doi: 10.3389/fpubh.2017.00008.

5. P. Horobin. "Male vs Female Pelvis." Peter Horobin Saddlery. Last modified 1 May 2015. https://horobin.com.au/journal/male-vs-female-pelvis.

6. D. Bennett. *Who's Built Best to Ride?* Livingston, CA: Equine Studies Institute, 2008. www.equinestudies.org/whos_built_best_2008/whos_built_best_2008_pdf1.pdf.

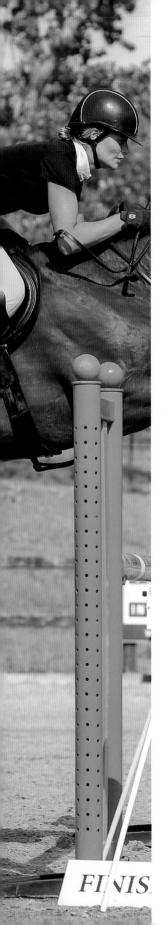

CHAPTER 2

Your Fascia

■ WHAT IS YOUR FASCIA?

It used to be thought that the fascia was a white filmy covering that surrounded the organs and muscles, holding them in place. This has now proved to be incorrect, and I am very excited to be working as part of the fast-growing world of fascia therapy, which is being backed up by many new strands of research.

Your fascia, or connective tissue, is a three-dimensional network of microscopic hollow tubules that joins every one of your cells together. This web is continuous with a network of fibers within each cell that connects with the nucleus. So there is no part of your body that is not connected to every other part via your connective tissue.

This continuity is nicely illustrated in this photo of half a lemon. You can see that the lemon is made up of different parts—the skin, pith, segments, and the pulps (containing the juice)—which have different functions. But at no point is there any separation between the parts, making up a continuous system with differentiated areas.

The fascia is mainly made up of:

* collagen fibers within the tubules, which give you strength and stability
* elastin fibers within the tubules to allow flexibility
* the ground substance that sits between your cells and fibers.

The gel-like ground substance is made up of water, hyaluronic acid,

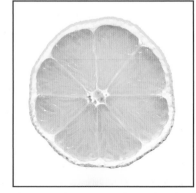

Photograph courtesy of @zcalvertl via Twenty20.

and proteoglycans. It provides the correct environment for your cells to function properly and allows the fibers to move and glide over each other, changing with the stresses and strains that are put on your body.[1]

In healthy conditions the fascial system is relaxed, providing strength, shape, flexibility, protection, and shock absorption, allowing you to move safely without restriction or pain. It is very strong, yet highly flexible and dynamic, adapting the position of the fibers depending on the stresses and strains put on it.[2]

But the ground substance solidifies in response to trauma—for example, a sudden impact—or over time if there is constant irritation, such as a repetitive movement. This is a very similar reaction to cornstarch or corn flour—when you mix it with water to the right consistency it becomes a non-Newtonian liquid. This means that it behaves like a liquid at times and a solid at other times. Jello and ketchup are other examples of things that react in this way.

When your ground substance solidifies the cells can't function correctly, which may lead to disease and inflammation, and the fibers are unable to adapt to change, so they tighten up, leading to pain and tension. This in turn causes restrictions in other parts of the body, creating abnormal pressure. This crushing pressure affects the nerves and blood and lymphatic vessels, and further increases the tension in pain-sensitive structures. It also makes you more prone to injury. Symptoms such as pain, stiffness, tingling, and numbness may be due to this.

When you are riding, it is your fascia that enables you to sit correctly, move in the way that you want when you want, and to feel and respond to what your horse is doing.

■ BIOTENSEGRITY

Architect and inventor Buckminster Fuller first talked about tensegrity in the 1970s, coining the term by combining the words "tension" and "integrity."

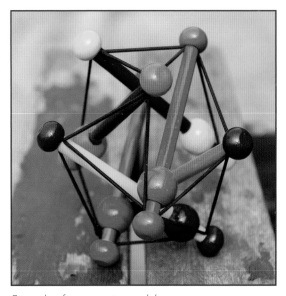

Example of a tensegrity model.

A tensegrity model is a structured system where the forces that compress it and those that put it under tension are balanced out. So changing any part of the system will have an effect on all the other parts. As you can see in this photo, if you were to cut one of the elastics or break one of the sticks, the whole structure would collapse. But when they are all intact and working as they should do, then the model is very strong, but flexible. Then, if you imagine a knot in one of the elastics, pulling it shorter, you can see that the sticks it is attached to will also be pulled. This in turn will alter the position of the other ends of those sticks, and pull on the elastics at those ends, and so on.

When this system is seen in biological structures, including humans, it is called biotensegrity.

Graham Scarr describes the human anatomy as a "network of structures under tension and others that are compressed; parts that pull things together and others that keep them apart."[3]

This system enables your body to adapt in a simple, efficient way to cope with forces that are potentially damaging. But once you add in scar tissue or other restrictions, they change that balance between tension and compression. Then, just like with the tensegrity model, the pull from the damaged part of your body will change the position and dynamics of every other part.

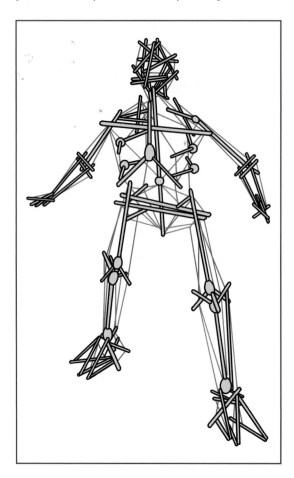

response to the stresses and strains put onto you, without losing your shape and structure.

Traditional models of medicine tend to focus on your skeleton, describing the bones as the fundamental load-bearing structures, into which all the muscles attach. Our understanding of biotensegrity tells us that actually your bones are merely the levers, and it is your fascial system that gives you your shape. This is such a different way of thinking about how our bodies are structured and how they work that it has been quite slow to be taken up by the medical profession. But, slowly, the research is spreading and the profession is beginning to look at bodies from a different perspective, just like my vases in the introduction.

Dr. Jean-Claude Guimberteau is a French hand surgeon who has led the way in recording and researching the architecture of the myofascia. His images beautifully show the continuity of the fibers and how they are able to respond to changes in their environment and the forces acting on them. He describes how the system is "mobile, can move quickly and interdependently, and is able to adapt its plasticity."[4]

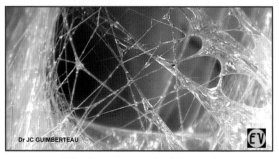

An image of the fascial network, showing the interconnectedness of the fibers. Photograph courtesy of Dr. J.-C. Guimberteau.

Biotensegrity is starting to explain how living systems are able to store energy for movement while maintaining stability. This property of your body is what allows you to move and change in

There are no straight lines in your body; all the different parts that work so brilliantly together to make the whole that becomes you are based on spiral shapes, fractals, and branches, which are found everywhere in nature. The Romanesco cauliflower in this photo demonstrates this property beautifully.

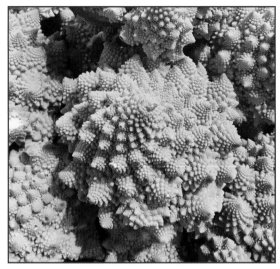

Photograph courtesy of @lfusco via Twenty20.

We are very used to seeing these beautiful repeating patterns in nature, but the idea that we are also made up in the same way is very new to most of us. But when you are aware of it, you can see bodies in a completely different light. The biotensegrity model explains that all your movements come from the interaction of repeated shapes within your body at all levels.

Your horse is the same—have a look at it moving and you will see that the patterns of movement that are made by the groups of muscles working together are quite beautiful. And if there is an area that doesn't seem to be flowing in the same way, it is probably the site of an old trauma or compensation that needs releasing.

■ HOW YOUR FASCIAL SYSTEM AFFECTS YOUR RIDING

If you had no restrictions within your fascial system, your body would have the ability to come back to its ideal position; even it was put under strain by trauma or repetitive movements, it would be able to spring back once the strain was removed.

But horses have fascia too!

Just as your body is constantly adapting to the stresses and strains put upon it, so is your horse's. Even before you put tack on and mount your horse, its body has fascial restrictions that may be causing pain and tightness that you are not aware of. The weight of the horse has to be distributed between its four feet. Ideally this would be an even distribution, but it is unlikely to be putting twenty-five percent of its weight through each foot owing to compensations for old injuries, the way it has been ridden, and even how it was born.

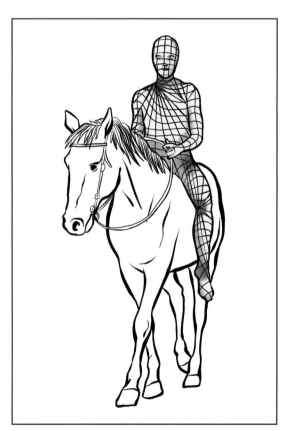

Fascia man on horse: how restrictions can affect your whole body.

When you are sitting on your horse's back, you have three points of contact—your seat through the saddle, and both feet through the stirrups. This is the position in which you have the most chance of equal weight distribution. But think about how this has to change during rising trot, jumping, or riding without stirrups. The more points of contact you have with your horse, the more your weight is distributed over its body and down through its legs. So every time you move your weight off and onto the horse, or even just shift your position, it has to change its own center of gravity.

Both of you are dealing with the effects of gravity separately and in your own ways, feeling what is going on in your own bodies, except you are now actually one unit with only four feet between you and the ground.

When you think about it like that, isn't it amazing that horses are able to perform such intricate dressage maneuvers and jump such incredible heights, all while compensating for our twists and torsions, as well as their own?

All the fibers of your fascial system, which are connecting every cell in you and in your horse, are continually adjusting, and not just in the parts of your body that are in contact with each other. So if your horse is being worked unevenly (by your body or schooling) it will develop lines of tension that will change how it moves. Whether you simply enjoy trail rides or you compete in barrel racing, these effects still apply to you and your horse every time that you ride.

In this way, you can see that if you are riding with pain, tension, or imbalances in your body,

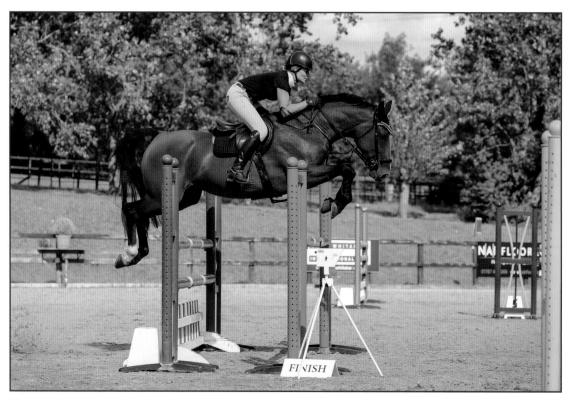

Photograph courtesy of Spencer Moret.

there will be an increased chance of injury and decreased performance in your horse. Just like human athletes, competition horses often suffer from repeated injuries in the same area of their body. This could be because of poor rehabilitation or going back to work too early, but it could also be linked to their riders having the same issues as before, going back to riding in the same way and putting the same forces through their horse's body.

If you are doing exercises to get fit again, it is important to use your muscles in the position that they will be put under stress in the future. If you are trying to get back to horse riding, there is no point in doing exercises only lying down. Your fascial system needs to be able to respond to the loads that will be put onto it. So, your exercise program should include functional work in sitting, to allow your system to develop in the correct way for your lifestyle.

■ REFERENCES

1. L. Chaitow and J. DeLany. *Clinical Application of Neuromuscular Techniques*. Vol. 1, *The Upper Body*. 2nd ed. Philadelphia, PA: Churchill Livingstone, 2008.
2. R. Schliep, T. W. Findley, L. Chaitow, and P. A. Huijing, eds. *Fascia: The Tensional Network of the Human Body*. Philadelphia, PA: Churchill Livingstone, 2012.
3. G. Scarr. *Biotensegrity: The Structural Basis of Life*. Pencaitland, Scotland: Handspring, 2014.
4. J.-C. Guimberteau. *Architecture of Human Living Fascia*. Pencaitland, Scotland: Handspring, 2015.

CHAPTER 3

How Your Body Reacts to Injury

Please remember that the advice given in this chapter is general in nature and if you require individual advice, you should consult your own therapist.

■ PHYSICAL REACTION

Your entire fascial network is continually responding to your environment, adapting to the stresses and strains that it is subjected to. This is its function: absorbing shock and flexing with the forces that are applied. But these changes should only be temporary, to allow your system to survive the injury, and then your fascia should gradually come back to its normal, relaxed state.

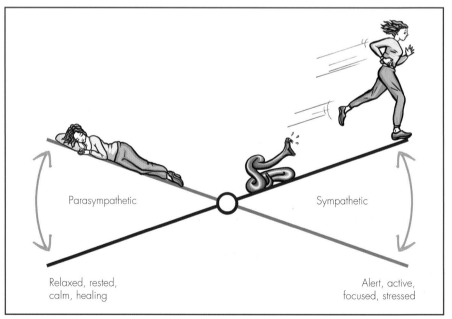

Parasympathetic		Sympathetic
Relaxed, rested, calm, healing		Alert, active, focused, stressed

The autonomic nervous system.

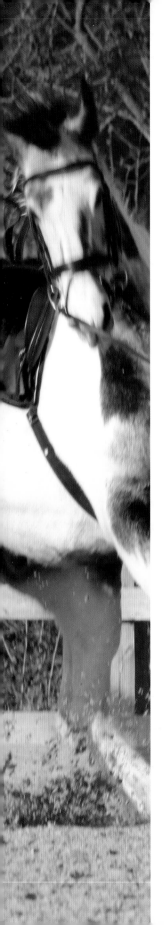

So, in normal conditions your body should be able to fully relax when you are resting but be ready to instantly spring into action if you are in danger. This balance is managed by your autonomic nervous system, which regulates your body's functions without you needing to have conscious control of them. There are two parts of the autonomic nervous system, which between them balance the reactions of your internal organs to your environment.

The sympathetic nervous system is stimulated when you are in danger (or perceived danger) and this is what produces the fight-or-flight response. That is when your adrenal glands release hormones, including adrenaline and cortisol, preparing your body for whatever it has to do to survive the dangerous situation. This has the effect of increasing your heart rate and blood pressure, expanding the air passages in your lungs, enlarging your pupils, and sending more blood to your muscles. This may save your life in an emergency, as you can find increased strength to defend yourself and improved reaction times.

The parasympathetic nervous system has the role of conserving and restoring. It regulates your organs under normal conditions, and, after danger has passed, it slows your heart rate and decreases your blood pressure. It also stimulates your digestive system to allow energy from food to heal and build your tissues. That is why people very often hear their tummy rumbling during a relaxing treatment.

The psoas muscle, also known as the fight-or-flight muscle, is one of your core muscles and you have one on each side. They run from the front of your hips through your pelvis, and attach to the front of your lower spine. These muscles are responsible for a lot of people's back pain and stiffness.

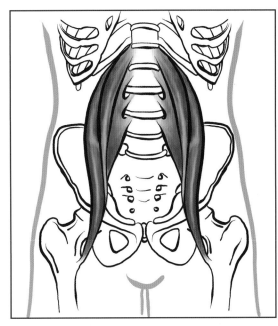

The psoas muscles.

Their main action is to flex your hips, but they also help to stabilize the base of your spine. Psoas is the only muscle that connects your trunk to the lower part of your body and passes from the front to the back of your body.

When you are stressed, in a dangerous situation, or have physical trauma, your sympathetic nervous system causes the psoas muscles to tighten. This protective response should only last for a couple of hours at the most, but for many people the tension is never released and it becomes normal to them.[1]

The protective fetal position that anxiety throws your body into causes a flexed posture, where your upper body is tipped forward and your center of gravity is further forward. If this happens when you are riding, the shift in your weight can overload the front of your horse.

Another trauma response that is less recognized is the freeze or immobility response. This is a very primitive reaction, which is better known in the animal world. Think of a mouse that has been hunted by a cat. Even if it has not been badly injured, it will become immobile while the cat is still around. This survival instinct is to give it the best chance of escaping if the cat gets bored and becomes distracted by something more interesting. But if the poor mouse remains the focus of attention and the cat tosses it around and then eats it, the immobility response keeps it in what Peter Levine calls an "altered state of consciousness," where it will feel no pain or awareness of suffering.[2]

If an animal (especially a prey animal in the wild) survives the dangerous event or a potential threat, it does not just carry on as though nothing has happened. It will go through a period of intense shaking once the danger has passed, to burn off the excess energy that has been released. Once this has been completed its system can return to normal, and it is unlikely to carry that trauma with it in the future. It will go through this cycle many times a day without long term ill effects, by simply following its body's natural reactions.

My dog has a shake after every time she pulls on the leash and her collar tightens. She is not in pain, but the tension that has come into her system needs releasing. How many times a day would your tension need to be released?

Owing to our ability to override this primitive reaction, our bodies retain the cell memory of the trauma and we have to compensate for that as long as it remains. Over our lifetimes, each frozen memory is layered onto the previous traumas, until we feel that we are encased in concrete. Then the fibers of our fascial system are unable to move and change as they need to, our cells cannot function as they should, and we end up with pain and disease.

This is why you often see athletes with the same injury over and over again. The layers of compensation make it very difficult to fully recover from traumas, and the tension created by each new incident joins the old holding patterns in your body.

Horse riders go through many potential and actual traumatic incidents, many of which may not be registered or acknowledged as being dangerous. The times when your horse has tried to take off across the field before you have managed to unclip the lead rope, but you regain control and everything is OK. Or when you are out for a quiet ride and your horse suddenly spooks for no apparent reason. Or how about the time when you thought that you were going to fall off, but saved yourself and stayed on. Each time that you feel that shot of adrenaline through your system, your body has recorded the exact position of each of your cells in that moment. Your subconscious will then try to protect you from going through the same thing again by avoiding that position. No wonder we get so stiff!

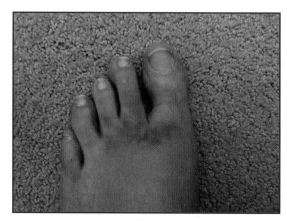

Photograph courtesy of @lksather via Twenty20.

Apart from falls, riders can have bruises, cuts, and sprains from their horses kicking, shoving, shying, and bolting. The jobs that need doing every day on the yard can also cause injuries other than the most common symptom of back pain. Walking into wheelbarrow handles and being trodden on by their horse seem to be frequent injuries among my patients. Most injuries from horse riding do not require a trip to hospital, but there are also a lot of injuries that go on to cause long-term pain, and other problems that never receive treatment.

■ EMOTIONAL RESPONSE

Many of us live in a permanent state of fight or flight; possibly because of previous traumas, or the stresses of everyday modern life. If our system is already on high alert, it does not take much in the way of extra stress to tip us over the edge into full-blown panic or meltdown.

As explained in the previous sections, your system carries tissue and cell memory. This does not record only past physical traumas, but the associated emotions too. This is why some situations instantly catapult us back to old memories, feelings, or reactions.

For example, I once treated a patient with a very deep scar on the side of his thigh from a bad accident. As soon as I touched the scar, he began to sweat and to feel extremely nauseous and anxious. Then he told me that after the surgery to repair his bone, which was nearly fifty years previously, his bone had become infected and he was extremely ill afterward. Even though the infection and bone had healed many years ago, the trauma of that time was still held within the fascia of this scar tissue.

If you have suffered a trauma, your fascial system and subconscious mind will have recorded the position that you were in at that point. Your mind then associates that particular position with danger or pain, so it will try to avoid it as much as possible. Have you ever noticed that some movements have a funny kink in them, or that if you try to do a certain movement it doesn't feel safe, so you just don't do it?

As far as your mind is concerned, the danger that you are reacting to doesn't have to have actually happened. You know that feeling when you think that the truck is going to hit your car? Or when you are riding and your horse suddenly spooks and you think that you are going to be thrown? The shot of adrenaline that flies through your system at that moment when you think that you are going to get seriously hurt is as real as the adrenaline that is released when you are actually injured.

You might have noticed it with your horse, too, as horses have the same reactions as us, but magnified as they are prey animals. So the horse that gets stressed when being loaded might be reacting to its tissue memory of a time years ago when it was hurt or scared in a similar situation.

In this way, old injuries and traumas (physical or emotional) lead to compensations that can affect you every day of your life. So it doesn't take much to shift your body from just about coping into spasm, pain, and inflammation. The thing that pushes you over your limit is often stress.

Stress has become the normal state for many of us, and over time it has an effect on your mind and body. Your brain interprets the tension as a sign of danger, and keeps the sympathetic nervous system on high alert. This cycle of chronic stress can lead to pain, tightness, fatigue, and breathing and digestive problems. Your fight-or-flight response is only meant to be in place for a couple of hours or days at the most. However, a lot of people are living in a permanent state of fight or flight, which affects their physical and emotional health.

If your stress response continues, it stops being helpful and can damage your health, immunity, mood, and quality of life, adding to the feelings of stress and anxiety. Then it is quite easy to trigger an extreme reaction like a panic attack or hyperventilation. It may also result in phobias.

Consider the stress cycle shown in the illustration—is this pattern familiar to you?

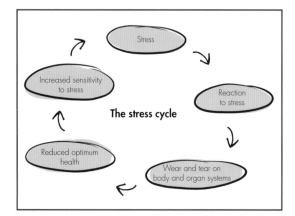

The stress cycle

This chain of events often leads to chronic pain and conditions such as fibromyalgia and chronic fatigue syndrome. It is the restrictions that are held in your fascial system that cause the reactions that lead to tension and the resulting physical and emotional illness.

▪ HOW TO HELP YOURSELF

- Identify your stress triggers and try to change or manage them.
- Even if you can't alter the situation, changing your reaction to it can still help.
- Set aside regular relaxation time.
- Exercise regularly, even it is just going for a walk.
- Eat a healthy diet.
- Get plenty of sleep.

- Find a local yoga or tai chi class and use the moves yourself every day.
- Learn mindfulness or meditation as a way of managing your daily stress.
- Accept the things that you can't change.

If you have a panic attack

A panic attack is when your body exaggerates its normal response to fear. They can be very frightening but cannot harm you physically or mentally. According to the *No Panic* website, common symptoms are:

- breathing difficulties
- pains or tightness of the chest
- palpitations
- feeling unreal or not there
- dizziness
- trembling
- sweating
- feeling faint or loss of balance
- a fear of not being in control
- a feeling that you can't cope
- a feeling of being trapped
- a feeling of losing control.[3]

If you feel that a panic attack is starting, there are a few things that you can do to reduce the feelings and calm things down:

- Breathe out slowly: Your natural reaction to stress is often to keep trying to breathe in but forgetting to breathe out first, so you end up with a lungful of stale air.
- Check your posture: Are you hunched over with your shoulders up around your ears? This position feeds back to your brain that you are under stress, even if you are not.
- Don't fight or run away from your symptoms—they will not harm you and

accepting them will help you to regain control faster.

- Remember that this is a normal reaction to stress and anxiety.
- If this is happening regularly, consider getting help from a trained professional who can help you to identify the reasons and work with you to reduce your reactions.

More help with how to breathe properly can be found in chapter 8.

■ FALLS

A few statistics:

- In the US, a study of horseback riders in three states showed that eighty-one percent were injured at some point in their career, twenty-one percent seriously. Novice riders were the most likely to be injured.[4]
- A UK report has suggested that one in five riders will be injured owing to a fall from a horse resulting in severe head or torso injuries.[5]

Even relatively minor falls cause an impact and affect your whole body via your fascial system, but if there is no major injury, falls are often ignored. The affect of the impact might not be in the part of the body that you landed on. The transmission of forces through your body should allow the shock of the impact to be distributed and not focused in one place. But old fascial restrictions block the shock and cause it to get stuck within the fascial network. This causes new restrictions on top of the old ones, and new symptoms to develop over time—separate from the immediate pain of the fall.

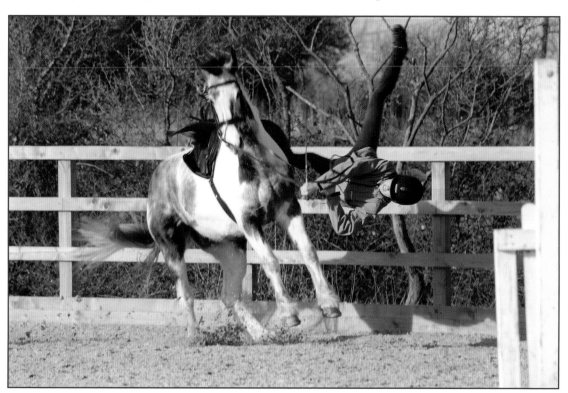

Photograph courtesy of Jess Morgan.

Your "normal" then becomes the tightness from old falls and injuries, as your brain gets used to it and stops telling you that there is a problem. Muscles can't work as effectively and can't be properly strengthened if they are tight and twisted. So the more impacts you have, the longer it will take to recover from injuries—and remember that impacts will affect your horse in the same way.

You may also tighten up and get a trauma response if you think you are going to fall, even if you don't. That is your protective mechanisms kicking in, as your sympathetic nervous system reacts to the perceived danger. So if you have had a near miss, try to give yourself time afterward to let go of any tension that you are still holding on to.

How to help yourself after a fall

- Even if you don't think that you were hurt, give yourself time to feel your body before you get back up. Remember the impact will affect your whole body, not just the part that you landed on or that is hurting.
- If you have been winded, don't panic. That feeling of not being able to take a proper breath can feel quite scary and that anxious feeling then makes it even harder to breathe. The reason that you can't breathe easily is that the impact makes your diaphragm (the main muscle that you use for breathing) go into spasm. Sit in a crouched position and try to take slow, deep breaths, remembering to give yourself time to breathe out before you breathe in again. If things do not improve after about fifteen minutes, seek medical attention to check that you do not have more serious injuries.
- If you have any bruises or swelling, rest the area initially, and then try to keep it moving gently. You may find that applying

a compression bandage helps to start with. For many years the advice was to use ice packs for injuries, but recently Dr. Gabe Mirkin, who originally gave that advice, has stated that using ice will delay healing and recovery.[6] This is because it narrows the blood vessels and limits the body's inflammatory response, which is essential for healing. He advises the use of ice packs for pain relief only in the first six hours after injury.

- Later in the day, try to gently stretch any tight areas, allowing your body to move as it needs to and not pushing into pain. For ideas on how to release specific areas, have a look at chapters 5 and 6.
- If you had any trauma to your head, make sure that you follow the guidelines below.

Concussion

Head injuries are starting to be taken seriously in many sports, including horse riding. The strict rules about wearing a hat that conforms to the latest safety recommendations have helped a lot, but most riders will be familiar with the feeling of their head bumping across the ground as they come to a halt after a fall (me included!).

It is therefore essential that riders and those caring for them are aware of the symptoms to look out for following a blow to the head, and what to do about it. These guidelines are from the US Equestrian Federation's concussion information page for horse riders:[7]

If any of these signs are observed following a head injury, the person should be checked by a health-care professional:

- Appears dazed or stunned
- Is unsure of whereabouts

- Moves clumsily
- Answers questions slowly
- Loses consciousness (even briefly)
- Shows behavior or personality changes
- Can't recall events before or after the fall
- Has a headache or feeling of pressure in head
- Is nauseous or vomiting
- Has balance problems or dizziness
- Has double or blurry vision
- Is sensitive to light or noise
- Has concentration or memory problems
- Feels sluggish or confused.

Even if you do not suffer with any of these symptoms, a blow to your head is a significant trauma and should be taken into consideration if you go on to suffer any other symptoms in the future.

■ REFERENCES

1. J. A. Staugaard-Jones. *The Vital Psoas Muscle*. Chichester, UK: Lotus, 2012.

2. P. Levine. *Waking the Tiger: Healing the Trauma*. Berkeley, CA: North Atlantic Books, 1997.

3. Silvermarbles. "Panic Attacks." No Panic. Last modified 22 July 2014. https://www.nopanic.org.uk/panic-attacks/.

4. C. Strickland. "Equine-Related Human Injuries." Horse: Your Guide to Equine Health Care. Last modified 1 October 2000. https://thehorse.com/14010/equine-related-human-injuries.

5. M. Chapman and K. Thompson. "Preventing and Investigating Horse-Related Human Injury and Fatality in Work and Non-work Equestrian Environments." *Animals (Basel)* 6, no. 5 (2016). doi:10.3390/ani6050033.

6. G. Mirkin. "Why Ice Delays Recovery." DrMirkin. 16 September 2015, last modified 2 May 2018. http://www.drmirkin.com/fitness/why-ice-delays-recovery.html.

7. US Equestrian Federation (USEF). "Heads Up Concussion." USEF. N.d., accessed 16 June 2018. https://www.usef.org/forms-pubs/b8tq8bEiaoM/heads-up-for-parents.

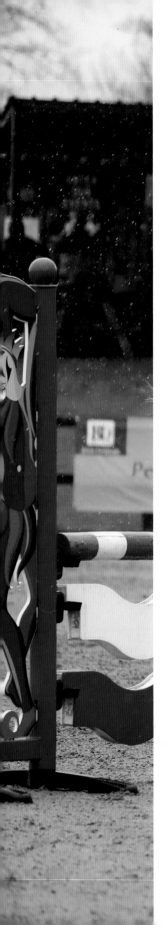

CHAPTER 4

Common Symptoms

Please remember that the advice given in this chapter is general in nature and if you require individual advice, you should consult your own therapist.

■ PAIN

A *British Medical Journal* report found that chronic pain affects between one-third and half of the population of the UK, which means that approximately twenty-eight million adults are living with pain.[1]

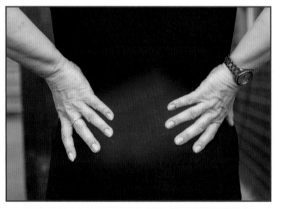

Pain is defined by the International Association for the Study of Pain as "an unpleasant sensory and emotional experience associated with actual or potential tissue damage, or described in terms of such damage."[2]

This means that the mind and body cannot be separated, and everyone's perception of pain is different. The amount of pain you feel doesn't only depend on how much damage you have sustained, but will vary according to what has happened to you in the past.

The pain felt after an injury is a necessary protective mechanism that makes you aware of the damage and ensures that you take action. It is a warning sign that needs to be acknowledged and responded to, not suppressed. But, in some people, this mechanism becomes stuck, leading to chronic or long-term pain.

You feel pain when the nerve endings that are sitting within your tissues are stimulated. There are receptors to pick up lots of different sensations, and some of them are specialized to sense those that may be harmful, such as heat, pressure, or chemicals. They communicate those sensations via your spinal cord to your brain, which is when you feel them. When those sensations reach a critical level, you will feel them as pain.

If the nerve endings in a certain area are overstimulated by constant irritation (such as pressure from the surrounding tissues or inflammation), even those that previously did not detect pain can become pain sensitive. It has been estimated that fascial restrictions put up to two thousand pounds per square inch of pressure on your nerve endings,[3] which is the equivalent of a fully grown draft horse sitting on you! This is how chronic pain (lasting more than three months) develops.

When the pain pathways from your nerve endings are stimulated, the receptors in your brain interpret this as your tissues being damaged and your brain sends painkilling chemicals to the area and triggers an inflammatory response and the repair process. This is essential when you actually have hurt yourself, but sometimes the cycle is continued not by a new injury, but by continued pressure on the nerve endings from your fascial restrictions.

The pain cycle can become an issue if an area is injured and then becomes swollen and inflamed, and the resulting tightness and scar tissue further irritates it. So the area never has a chance to settle and the nerve endings keep telling your brain that there is damage. So then the inflammation also becomes chronic, and the cycle keeps going around and around.

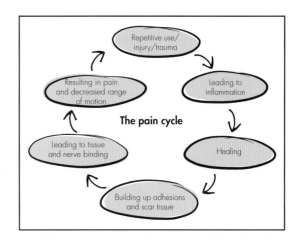

Chronic pain affects all areas of life as it can lead to lack of sleep, fatigue, irritation, depression, and anxiety. People's relationships and jobs suffer, and previously enjoyable activities such as horseback riding become difficult or even impossible.

Taking medication is the most common solution offered by doctors, but remember that the cause of your pain may be in a completely different part of your body to where you are feeling the symptoms. Medical investigations to find out if there is any cause of your pain that needs immediate treatment are essential, but medication can mask what you are feeling and does not necessarily address the root cause.

There are some environmental conditions that will make things harder for everyone, even those not living with constant pain. The weather is a big factor that can't be controlled, and prolonged spells of cold, wet weather will test even the most enthusiastic horse owner. Being prepared by having the right clothing and equipment is the best way to get through those long winters.

Using heated seats or hot packs in your car on the way to the yard—or even having a warm bath before you leave the house—will help your back to stay flexible, and at least you will start off feeling warm. You can also get heated patches that stick to your clothes, and these are particularly good for arthritic joints.

Do your joints let you know when damp, rainy weather is coming without you needing to see the forecast? According to a study done at Harvard Medical School, 67.9 percent of people surveyed felt the same.[4] It concluded that the increased pain may be due to a change in barometric pressure (atmospheric pressure), which normally pushes against the body from the outside. When the weather worsens, the barometric pressure falls, causing tissues in the body to expand and push on the nerve endings that signal pain.

■ TENSION

Why do you feel tight?

When your body is loose, relaxed and elastic, it can move and change with you. Over time it is very common to gradually feel tighter, but it isn't inevitable. My patients often tell me that they didn't realize their tightness was anything that could be changed as they have had it for so long. They blame themselves for not exercising, living with stress, and getting older.

There are several possible reasons for tension to build up in your tissues:

- **Dehydration:** The fibers in your fascial system (as described in chapter 2) need their environment to be fluid to allow them to move and adapt to the forces put on your body. If you are dehydrated, the fibers are less able to do this and they become stuck and locked down. You will feel this as knots in your muscles and stiffness around your joints.

- **Poor posture:** If you spend most of your time in positions that put your body under strain, it will react by tensing up to protect itself. For example, looking down for long periods of time will result in tension in the back of your neck.
- **Overusing muscles:** As with poor posture, putting your muscles under pressure when they are fatiguing will cause the fibers in the area to tighten up to protect the muscles.
- **Stress:** One of the hormones produced by your body in response to stress stimulates your kidneys to resorb water from your system, which can lead to dehydration.
- **Not stretching properly after exercise:** Muscles that have worked hard during exercise will naturally shorten as they cool down. If you do not create the conditions that allow them to open up again, that tension will remain.
- **Pain or weakness in a different part of your body:** This means that other areas of your body will need to work differently to compensate for the affected part not doing its job properly. The resulting imbalance causes tightness as muscles overwork.

As the pressure builds up in your muscles and they stiffen up, they gradually get thicker and shorter. This means that the blood flow isn't as good as it should be to help with healing, so you get more scarring, which makes the area even stiffer. Stretching opens up the layers of your muscles, helps the blood flow, and takes the pressure off the nerves. So pain and inflammation can be prevented or improved.

Remember that where you feel your symptoms is often different to where the cause of them is actually located. Your tightness may be due to problems in another part of your body and is your body's way of compensating and trying to protect itself. So there is no point in simply stretching the tight part without also finding and treating the cause. If the tension is not released it can become a holding pattern in your body that then has to be compensated for, adding to the cycle of tension.

Tension in your body makes it much harder for you to feel and respond to what your horse is doing. This applies when you are in the stall, leading, or doing ground work, as well as when you are riding. You will see in chapter 6 that many of the issues with riding position are either caused by or result in increased tension. It is then much harder to achieve a balanced seat with soft hands.

■ INFLAMMATION

Inflammation is defined as "redness, swelling, pain, and/or a feeling of heat in an area of the body. This is a protective reaction to injury, disease, or irritation of the tissues."[5]

Inflammation is an essential healing response that enables your body to respond to trauma, and is a sign that your body is reacting in the correct way to the injury. There are different stages of the inflammatory response, and they need to be completed for full healing to occur.

The signs of inflammation are:

- redness
- swelling
- tenderness
- increased temperature
- loss of function.

The stages of the inflammatory response are:

- **Stage 1:** This first, acute phase of healing lasts two to four days, when the aim is to start the healing process and to protect the area from further injury. The blood supply to the injured area increases, to bring chemicals and cells that help healing to the area, and to remove damaged cells. This is when you will feel the most pain, warmth, and swelling.
- **Stage 2:** The second, subacute phase lasts up to six weeks and is the repair phase of healing. Scar tissue is formed but is still weak and vulnerable to further injury. Your pain and swelling should start to reduce in this stage.
- **Stage 3:** The late, remodeling stage is between six weeks and three months after the initial injury. Your scar tissue begins to strengthen and become more organized in response to the loads that are put on it. This is when it is important to move the injured area as normally as possible so that your body can heal in the correct way for the function required. Your range of movement and strength will improve during this stage.

Anything beyond three months is the chronic phase, which can continue for months after the injury.

The inflammatory healing process can be interrupted if the area is under strain. This may come from fascial restrictions in other areas or from overuse before the injury has had time to heal sufficiently. If this continues and the inflammation becomes chronic, it may lead to chronic pain too, as explained earlier in this chapter.

Inflammation does not only occur following an injury, though. As with the delay in healing, if an area is constantly irritated by tension transmitted through your fascial system, your tissues react as though they have been injured. Then, if the cause of the irritation continues you will end up with chronic inflammation, which sometimes lasts for years.

This response is usually the root cause of conditions that seemingly appear for no reason, such as plantar fasciitis, tennis elbow, and bursitis. They will be resistant to local treatment for as long as the irritation persists.

■ REFERENCES

1. A. Fayaz, P. Croft, R. M. Langford, L. J. Donaldson, and G. T. Jones. "Prevalence of Chronic Pain in the UK: A Systematic Review and Meta-analysis of Population Studies." *BMJ Open* 6, no. 6 (2016): e010364. doi:10.1136/bmjopen-2015-010364.

2. H. Merskey and N. Bogduk. "Pain Terms: A Current List with Definitions and Notes on Usage." Part 3 in *Classification of Chronic Pain*, 2nd ed., International Association for the Study of Pain (IASP) Task Force on Taxonomy. Seattle: IASP, 1994.

3. K. Kayate. 1961. "The Strength for Tension and Bursting of Human Fasciae." *Journal of the Kyoto Prefectural Medical University* 1969 (1961): 484–88.

4. R. N. Jamison, K. O. Anderson, and M. A. Slater. "Weather Changes and Pain: Perceived Influence of Local Climate on Pain Complaint in Chronic Pain Patients." *Pain* 61, no. 2 (1995): 309–15.

5. PubMed Health. "Inflammation." PubMed Health Glossary. N.d., accessed 16 June 2018. https://www.ncbi.nlm.nih.gov/pubmedhealth/PMHT0022625/.

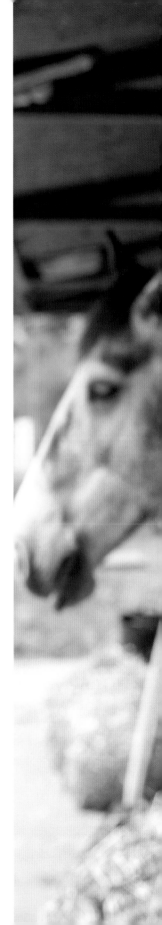

CHAPTER 5

Some Conditions Affecting Riders

The conditions listed here are just some of the more common problems experienced by riders, but of course there are many more. Some people are in constant pain in multiple areas while others might only ever have one problem.

Whatever you are feeling, please note that the advice given in this chapter is only a guide and can never replace medical assessment and treatment if that is what is required. So if you are unsure, or require individual advice, please do see your doctor or bodyworker. Remember that we each have our own medical history, which builds up to give the pattern of our symptoms over time. You could take ten people with identical symptoms and the cause and treatment would be different for each person. Because of this, the advice given here is very general, and it is essential to follow your own body and to trust what you feel.

Treating yourself: Research has shown that applying gentle, sustained pressure to an area for at least five minutes stimulates the body's anti-inflammatory response and so can speed healing.[1] Some of the advice given here is on how you can treat yourself using this method. Remember to go slowly and gently and to stop before you feel pain or if you experience any adverse effects.

■ BACK PAIN

According to the National Health Service in England (NHS England), back pain is the largest single cause of disability in the UK,[2] while a study of lower back pain in America found that seventy to ninety percent of the population are affected at some stage in their lifetime.[3]

Back pain can be a result of several different pathologies, and some people will have more than one problem contributing to their pattern of pain. These can include damage to muscles, tendons, ligaments, vertebral discs, and vertebrae.

Having said that, most back pain is not related to anything serious, and by keeping moving, avoiding aggravating tasks, and doing gentle exercise and stretches it should be possible to control it.

A recent article published in the *Lancet* examined the research into lower back pain assessment and treatment.[4] The conclusion was that there was very little evidence for most of the invasive investigations, X-rays, scans, injections, and surgeries. The authors did find that some manual therapy was helpful, together with a graded exercise program.

However, there are some "red flag" symptoms that may indicate a more serious problem. If you are experiencing any of these, it is very important to seek medical attention so that you can be checked and treated if necessary, especially if they come on following trauma such as a fall from your horse. The symptoms to look out for are:

- numbness or pins and needles between your legs, in the area that would be in contact with the saddle
- inability to pass urine
- urinary or bowel incontinence
- leg weakness
- extreme pain in both or one of your legs.

How your riding is affected

Horse riders are particularly vulnerable to back pain, which is commonly exacerbated by the jobs involved in looking after horses, and chapter 8 has a lot of advice on how to do jobs on the yard while taking care of your back. Studies have shown that the type of saddle used, stirrup length, and riding position all affect the incidence of lower back pain in riders.[5]

Horse riding itself can contribute to back pain too, and this is thought to be because of the compressive forces that are transmitted up through the rider's vertebral column. It can also cause your spine to move too far into flexion or extension, especially in sitting trot.[5]

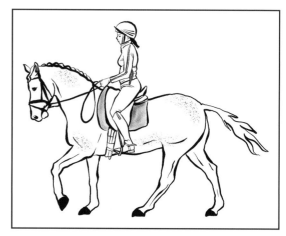

Position of the psoas muscles when riding.

As discussed in chapter 3, your psoas muscles are very important in stabilizing your lower back. As they attach directly into your spine, when they tighten up they cause pain and tension in your back. Even if the original cause of your pain is elsewhere, the psoas will tend to join in, making your symptoms worse. So it is always worth keeping the psoas released as well as treating whatever else is going on.

To be able to follow the rhythm of your horse's body when you are riding, your psoas muscles need to be able to alternately lengthen and shorten. So, if they are in a constantly shortened state, it will have the effect of jarring your horse's back too.

Intervertebral discs are the soft, gel-filled cushions that sit between each vertebra in your spine. They act as shock absorbers, while allowing safe movement of your spine. Spinal scans often report degenerative changes of the discs, or wear and tear. This is a natural change as you age and the water content of the discs reduces from the eighty percent that you are born with.

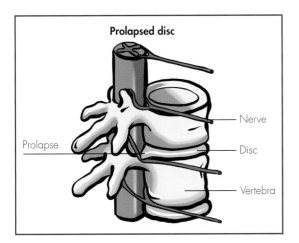

Prolapsed disc

Prolapse · Nerve · Disc · Vertebra

If a disc is compressed too much on one side—by trauma or muscle tension—the gel is forced out to the other side (imagine what would happen if you filled a balloon with water and then squeezed it on one side). This pushes part of the disc out of its normal position and into the space occupied by the nerves—a slipped disc—resulting in very painful conditions such as sciatica and nerve pain in your arms. When seeking treatment for disc problems, it is important to remember that even though your pain may be on one side, the cause is probably on the other side. Relieve the compression and the disc will have space to come back into its rightful position, as long as it has not completely ruptured or displaced too much.

How to help yourself

Psoas release with ball

Lie on your stomach on the floor. On whichever side of your lower back feels the loosest, locate the bone at the front of your pelvis. Don't worry

if you are not sure which side to start with, you will not do any damage by doing your tighter side first. Place the tennis ball up from the bone and toward your belly button. Lie face down on the ball for ten minutes, or as long as is comfortable. Repeat on the other side.

This release can also be done on a bed, but put a book under the ball so that it doesn't disappear into the mattress. Use pillows to keep your neck comfortable. Stop if any symptoms get worse.

Do not do this release if you are pregnant, think you might be pregnant, or have had recent abdominal surgery.

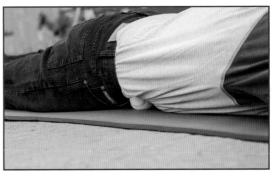

Psoas release with ball.

Spine release with foam roller

For the best results, this should be done regularly and you should aim to spend twenty to thirty minutes on it each time. If you feel this exercise is making any symptoms worse, stop.

Choose an area of floor with enough space for you to lie with your arms and legs spread out, and place the roller in the middle.

Sit on the edge of the roller and lower yourself down so your spine is along the length of it, with your head well supported. Keep your knees bent and your feet flat on the floor, and allow your arms to rest on the floor. Remain in this position until your body feels relaxed and completely comfortable. This may take the whole session—if this is the case, do not push your body further.

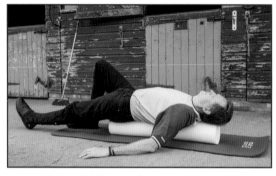

Spine release with foam roller.

If you feel able, slowly take your arms out to the side, keeping contact with the floor. Stop as soon as you feel pulling and before you feel pain. Remember you may feel things anywhere in your body, and your arms might need to be at different levels. Wait in the position that you feel the tightness until it releases. This will probably take a few minutes.

Do the same with your legs, but one at a time (otherwise you might fall off the roller!). Find a position of tightness and wait for the release. Please note that your body's requirements will be different every time you use your roller. Therefore, remember to follow your body—it doesn't matter how far you move, as long as you stop at the barriers.

If you find the roller too high for your back to be comfortable, try using a half roller instead.

Alternative releases:

- Chapter 5: Fibromyalgia—the constructive rest position

- Chapter 6: Lower back too arched—psoas release
- Chapter 6: Unable to straighten after dismounting—psoas release

■ NECK PAIN

Like your back, your neck can be affected by the muscles, tendons, joints, and ligaments in the area causing pain, and the pain will be made worse if you are doing anything that puts strain on it.

Often pain that is felt at the back of your neck is due to tension in the muscles at the front. This pulls your head and spine forward, with gravity also pushing down. So to stop yourself looking at the ground the whole time, the muscles at the back of your neck have to work harder to lift your head back into a more upright position.

If you have had any trauma to your head or neck and then you experience any of the following symptoms, it is important to get checked by a medical professional:

- Extreme pain in your neck or arms
- Dizziness
- Bad headache
- Weakness in one or both arms
- Urinary or bowel incontinence
- Difficulty controlling your legs when walking.

How your riding is affected

The main effect that neck pain has on your riding is due to the tension that is almost always associated with it. As your head is relatively heavy and riding requires you to be balanced, the muscles in your neck and upper back will tend to tense up to support your head and protect your neck.

The more you push your body while you have neck pain, the greater the protective response, and this will result in tension being transmitted into your shoulders and down your arms. So your horse will be able to sense your neck pain through the reins and in its mouth.

How to help yourself

Neck release with ball

Stand against a wall and position the ball at the back of your neck, just to the side of your spine. This can also be done with two balls at the same time, one on either side. Lean back onto the ball, slowly feeling it sink into your body until it meets resistance, then stop. Wait in that position, keeping the rest of your body soft, and feel as your muscles open up.

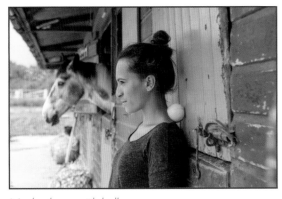

Neck release with ball.

For the best results, this release should take at least five minutes, but if you are very sore, you should follow your body and stop if you need to. Remember that you are not looking to find the painful spots, just resistance. If the ball is on a point that is sore, try readjusting it so you are more comfortable.

You could do this release while standing and leaning against a wall, sitting in a high-backed chair, or lying on your back on the floor or bed.

Alternative releases:

- Chapter 6: Chin forward
- Chapter 6: Shoulders elevated

■ TENDONITIS

The meaning of "-itis" is inflammation, so tendonitis is simply inflammation of a tendon. Tendons are the strong bands that attach each end of your muscles to bone. They are vulnerable to injury and inflammation because they are not very stretchy and do not have as good a blood supply as the muscle itself.

This means that if they are injured—for example, being overstretched or twisted or suffering a direct blow—it takes much longer for them to heal. Tendonitis can also occur when stress is put onto the tendon from tightness and restrictions elsewhere in your body. For instance, if your pelvis is rotated, the forces transmitted through your fascial network will put your muscles and tendons under tension. So if there is even a minor injury, the tendon is much more likely to overstretch and become inflamed. This may happen without an actual injury if the irritation from other restrictions is bad enough.

Tendonitis can affect any muscle, but the most common places are shoulders (rotator cuff disease), elbows (tennis and golfer's elbow), and ankles (Achilles tendonitis). More information about inflammation can be found in chapter 4.

How your riding is affected

Riding may aggravate your tendonitis because of the repetitive movements and positions that you need to be in. When a particular part of your body is painful, your subconscious reaction is to avoid the pain by shifting position or moving differently. This, of course, will alter your balance when you are riding, so other muscles will have to take over and work harder to allow you to keep going.

How to help yourself

Rest

Your body needs time to heal, and the inflammatory response is its way of healing. If you keep doing the things that are aggravating your tendon injury, your body will not have a chance to do its job and it will delay healing. There will always be jobs that have to be done, but if it is possible to get help or to do them more slowly or in a different way than usual, you will be out of pain more quickly and less likely to suffer the long-term problems of chronic inflammation.

Gentle movement

It is important to keep moving to avoid the area becoming stiff. Common sense needs to be applied here! Don't worry about moving the area, but do not push into pain.

Treat yourself

To do this for yourself, gently put one hand over the affected tendon, allow it to sink into the skin and wait. No need to push or try to move anything—the warmth and pressure from your hand will also help your ground substance to become more fluid, and the fibers will start to release. Stop if it doesn't feel right, if it is uncomfortable to maintain the position, or if it is painful.

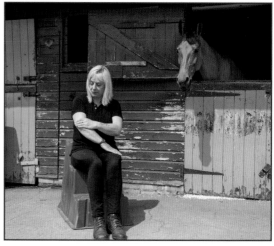

Treating yourself.

■ FIBROMYALGIA

Fibromyalgia is a chronic condition that causes widespread pain and fatigue. Sufferers often also report muscle stiffness and increased sensitivity. As this condition presents differently in each person and does not have a definitive diagnostic test at the moment, diagnosis is dependent on your doctor being aware of the condition and its implications.

Ginevra Liptan is an American doctor who also has fibromyalgia, and she now specializes in treating and researching the condition. Her excellent book *The FibroManual* has a lot of information, and if you are interested in finding out more I would recommend reading this and following her on social media as she regularly publishes updates on the latest research.

How your riding is affected

Although some fibromyalgia sufferers have to stop riding altogether for at least a period of time, there are many who find that riding is beneficial to their general well-being. This is a condition that is worsened by stress, so finding a low-impact, enjoyable form of exercise that releases endorphins and helps to strengthen your core muscles is invaluable. The compromises are often in the kind of riding that you are able to do, as fast-paced and endurance rides are more likely to cause problems.

How to help yourself

The Constructive Rest Position

This is a yoga pose that focuses on allowing your lower back and particularly the psoas muscles to relax. It is a neutral position that reduces muscle tension and can even help to clear your mind. It is beneficial if you have fibromyalgia because of the link between the psoas and your autonomic nervous system, which can affect energy levels and sensitivity to pain.

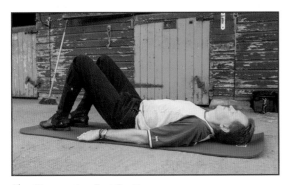

The Constructive Rest Position.

- Lie on your back with your knees bent and your feet on the ground. Your feet should be in line with your seat bones and far enough away from each other to allow your knees to rest against each other.
- You may need a small pillow or towel under your head to support your neck.
- You can also have your legs raised and resting on a chair or pillows if that is more comfortable for you.
- Your arms can rest on the floor or on your tummy, whichever you find most relaxing.
- Then do nothing.
- Focus on your breathing: four counts in, pause, six counts out. This will help your whole body to relax and let go.
- Do this for ten to twenty minutes a day if you can, remembering to follow your body and build up slowly if you need to. If you have time, longer sessions are advisable or even two sessions a day.

The advice in chapter 8 is very helpful for managing the symptoms of fibromyalgia, especially the section on listening to your body.

Dr. Liptan's research has found that people with fibromyalgia show significant long-term benefits from Myofascial Release treatment.[6] Chapter 9 in this book has all the details on this treatment.

Alternative release:

- Chapter 7: At the end of the day

■ OSTEOARTHRITIS

Osteoarthritis is sometimes known as wear and tear or degeneration of a joint. It can occur in any joint of the body and is a result of either abnormal use of a normal joint or normal use of an abnormal joint. In other words, you are much more likely to develop osteoarthritis if you were born with congenital abnormalities, if you have ever injured the joint, or if the joint is used over and over again in the same way.

The bony ends that come together to form a joint are covered by a thin layer of cartilage that protects them and produces the joint fluid for lubrication. As the joint begins to degenerate, this layer is gradually worn away so there is less lubrication and more friction between the bone ends. Severe arthritis is when there is very little cartilage left and the bone ends themselves start to wear.

Osteophytes are areas of extra bone that the body lays down to try to repair the damage done by the arthritis. They are normally on the outside of joints and look like nodules. They can cause a lot of pain as they push on nerves in the area and lead to inflammation.

Typical symptoms are stiffness if you haven't moved for a while, especially first thing in the morning, and pain which gets worse if you do too much. You can also get swelling around the affected joint and tightness in the surrounding muscles.

How your riding is affected

Riders typically suffer from arthritis in their hips, knees, spine, and fingers. This is probably because of the repetitive movements in riding and poor manual handling techniques when doing jobs round the yard. Chapter 7 has lots of suggestions on how to change these.

As with other painful conditions, it is the tension around the joint that causes most of the problems when you are riding. This is because your other muscles need to work differently to maintain your balance and this compensation is felt by your horse, which will then also need to compensate and change its movements.

How to help yourself

Regular movement

Movement will prevent the joint from stiffening up and it will also feel less painful when you start to move if it hasn't had a chance to seize up in one position. Gentle exercise will not be damaging to an arthritic joint, even if it feels a bit sore to start with. As long as you are following what you feel and not forcing it into any positions, moving will be helpful.

Strengthening exercises for the muscles around the joint

Most joints rely on the muscles around them for support, but if a joint is painful you are less likely to move it so the muscles can weaken quite quickly. There are many variations of exercises that can be suitable but it is important that you are assessed and then advised by a professional who can give you the exercises that are right for you.

Find a practitioner who can give you treatment to release the soft tissue around the joint and take the strain off it, to allow for reduction in inflammation and to prevent worsening of the arthritis.

JOINT PAIN AND STIFFNESS

■ HAND AND WRIST PAIN AND STIFFNESS

Common reasons for hand and wrist problems are arthritis, tendonitis, carpal tunnel syndrome, and fractures or dislocations of the fingers.

How your riding is affected

Whatever the cause, pain and stiffness in your hands is like torture to a horse rider, being aggravated by every job and by riding itself. So many riders live with this pain and push on through when they don't have to. There are simple changes that you can make that will help your hands to cope with the jobs you need them to do:

* **Keep them warm and dry:** Wearing a good pair of thermal gloves can make a huge difference to how your hands react to winter weather. This does sound really obvious, but I have seen people only think about putting on gloves once their fingers have gone numb and the joints are stiff. Prevention is much less painful! Disposable heat pads for gloves are great.
* **Keep releasing them:** Most of the jobs on the yard involve gripping, and that is before you have to hold the reins. So as soon as you become aware of your fingers and hands tightening up, pause what you are doing, wriggle your fingers, circle your wrists, and stretch your hand gently open.

How to help yourself

Hand-on-ball release

Sit in a comfortable position with your shoulders relaxed. Rest your hand over the top of a tennis ball or one of similar size, on a flat surface. Gently start to roll the ball under your hand but keep your fingers relaxed—they shouldn't be gripping the ball at all. If you feel that the rolling movement slows or stops, rest and wait in that position, allowing the weight of your hand to sink onto the ball.

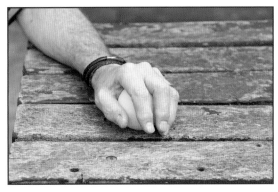

Hand-on-ball release.

Once the restriction softens and releases, you will easily be able to roll on the ball again until the next stop. It may take a few minutes for the tightness to release but it is worth being patient and waiting for it to change properly. The idea of this exercise is to find and feel the tight areas, which will be in different places each time you do it. Never push into pain—if a spot is very tender, just roll off it slightly so that you can release the tissue around the painful area.

Finger pulls

This is a great way for you to treat yourself that can be done anywhere (even when sitting on your horse). Each of your fingers has three joints, which can all be affected by pain and stiffness. By gently releasing the soft tissues around the joints, you will increase the blood flow to the area and take the strain off the joint. You can do this for all of your fingers if you find that both your hands tighten up if you are gripping for a long time, or working in the cold. Or if you only have one or two affected fingers, it is fine to do the self-treatment just on them.

Rest your arm in a comfortable position, then gently hold the finger that you are going to treat between the thumb and first finger of your other hand. Very slowly start to apply a gentle traction to your finger, without moving over the skin. It is very important to stay focused so that you can feel as soon as you feel a resistance to the pull. Never pull into pain. Once you have found the tightness, maintain the traction until you feel your finger soften or lengthen. Then slowly release your pull and move on to the next finger as needed.

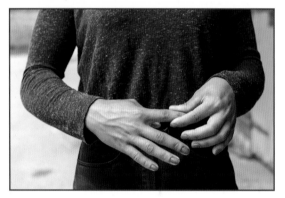

Finger pull.

Alternative release:

♦ Chapter 6: Gripping your reins too hard

▪ ELBOW PAIN AND STIFFNESS

Elbow pain is often due to tendonitis and is in response to ongoing tension and irritation. If it is the outer edge of your elbow that is sore, it is known as tennis elbow, and pain on the inner edge is called golfer's elbow.

Another cause of elbow pain is arthritis, as described earlier in this chapter. Often it is secondary to an old injury such as a fracture or dislocation, especially if surgery was needed at the time. Elbow injuries can be very problematic to heal and people can be left with stiffness for the rest of their lives.

If patients tell me about trauma to their elbow in the past, I have come to expect that they will not be able to straighten it fully and to be a bit stiff and sore at the end of trying to bend it. Most of the time they have come to see me about a completely different part of their body as they just live with the pain and inconvenience of their old injury.

How your riding is affected

Riders have told me that their elbows get very painful when they are mucking out, lifting buckets of water, raking, and poo picking. This pain may be due to any of the above reasons, but you do not necessarily have to live with it.

How to help yourself

Elbow release

Straighten your arm out in front of you as far as is comfortable, with your palm facing downwards. Let your wrist relax so your hand drops down, and then use your other hand to very gently increase the stretch until you feel a pull into your forearm. Do not stretch into pain though.

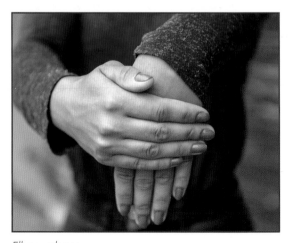

Elbow release.

Hold that gentle pull until you feel it soften and ease up, then bring your hand back to neutral. Next, keeping your arm straight, bend your wrist up so your hand moves toward the ceiling and hold at the point that you feel a gentle pull, until it releases.

Get your neck and back checked

Most of the patients that I see with elbow pain have had a lot of different treatments and interventions, all to the elbow, and mostly with only temporary benefit. That is because some of the muscles attaching into your elbow link up to your shoulder. Tension in your back and neck is very easily transferred into your shoulders and down your arms, irritating the tendons in your elbows and causing inflammation.

Alternative releases:

* Chapter 5: Tendonitis
* Chapter 6: Elevated shoulders

■ SHOULDER PAIN AND STIFFNESS

Shoulder problems typically present as pain and stiffness in and around the joint and are given different labels depending on the exact nature of the symptoms. In my experience, shoulder symptoms are normally connected to other areas of your body, even if there has been direct trauma to the shoulder joint. Your body should be able to heal injuries and inflammation so if you are left with a chronic problem, the reason for it should be looked for elsewhere in your body. For example, your pelvis might be out of alignment or you may have scar tissue holding on to surrounding tissues.

How your riding is affected

Riding with shoulder pain is not only very uncomfortable, but the resulting tension also puts strain on your arms, hands, neck, and back.

How to help yourself

Shoulder circles

Cradle the elbow on your sore side in your opposite hand, completely relaxing your arm. Using your good arm and starting small, take your elbow round in gradually increasing circles.

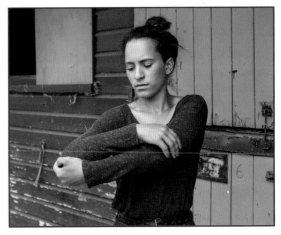

Shoulder circles.

Do not push into painful areas, but if you feel resistance and the feeling that it will become painful if you keep going, rest at that point. Keep your elbow relaxed into your hand until you feel it soften. Then you can repeat and find other points of tension.

Alternative releases:

* Chapter 6: One shoulder further forward
* Chapter 6: Elevated shoulders

■ KNEE PAIN AND STIFFNESS

The knee joint is very complex and is prone to injury and inflammation. Some common problems are arthritis, tendonitis, bursitis, ligament injuries, patella (knee cap) problems, and torn cartilage. Your knees often suffer from the strain put on them if your pelvis is out of alignment or if the muscles around your hips are tight.

The problem with most knee conditions is that because it is difficult to avoid the painful positions or movements, your body very quickly starts to compensate. Your knee joint relies a lot on your quadriceps (thigh) muscles to support it, but this group of muscles weakens relatively quickly if not used properly. You will know if this is happening to you if your thigh tires quickly and your knee gives way suddenly.

How your riding is affected

Riders with knee pain often find it difficult to support themselves through their left knee when mounting, finding a comfortable length to have the stirrups, and going through the constant bending and straightening of rising trot.

How to help yourself

Quadriceps exercises

Your knee is reliant on the strength of the muscles around it to support and stabilize the joint. So maintaining good quadriceps muscle strength is very important. These exercises need to be taught face to face, as the person teaching you needs to check that you are doing them correctly. If your knees ever give way or

lock, see your doctor for tests and a referral to a therapist who is qualified to assess and treat you.

Thigh release with ball

Facing a wall, place the ball at the front of your thigh, just below your hip. Then lean into the wall so that you feel gentle pressure from the ball, but no pain. Wait in that position until you feel your muscle soften, then move the ball down to the next tight area and repeat.

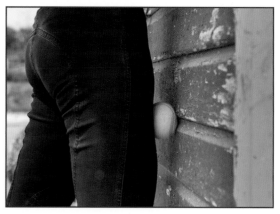

Thigh release with ball.

This release can also be done using a foam roller against the wall, or lying on your front on the floor or bed with the ball or roller under your thigh. Both thighs can be released at the same time with one roller or two balls.

Alternative release:

♦   Chapter 6: Lower back too arched

■ HIP PAIN AND STIFFNESS

Your hips are particularly susceptible to inflammation and tightness as they are directly articulating with your pelvis. As you will realize by now, if your pelvis has rotated and fixed in that position, your whole body has to compensate. But this is especially true of your hip joints and the soft tissue around them. Common hip problems include arthritis, bursitis, and tendonitis.

The tendonitis occurs because all the muscles in the area come under a lot of strain when the bones into which they are attaching are in the wrong position. The muscles that mainly affect your hips are your quadriceps (at the front of your thighs), hamstrings (at the back of your thighs), pelvic floor, and tensor fascia lata. This muscle is mostly made up of tendon and is more commonly known as the ilio-tibial band or IT band. It is the tight band that runs down the outside of your thighs.

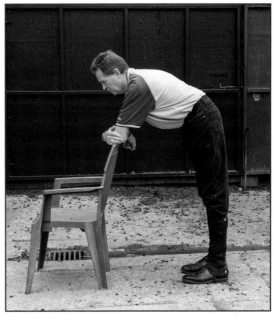

Hamstring release.

How your riding is affected

All aspects of riding will be affected by hip pain and stiffness: from mounting and dismounting to simply sitting on your horse, and controlling your body in all the paces. This problem at the center of your body will then pull into other areas as they have to work harder to compensate. You will also often find that you are tighter in the side opposite to where the pain is the worst.

How to help yourself

Hamstring release

Lean forward and rest your upper body on the back of a chair or table. You may need to try different heights to find which works best for you. Lift your tailbone toward the ceiling and drop your lower back toward the floor, feeling for the release in the backs of your legs.

As the tissue releases, allow your body to shift forward, back, or to either side to access the next layer of restriction. Actively lower your back further toward the floor, while lifting your tailbone higher to increase elongation. Try with both legs together, or one leg at a time, with your non-weight-bearing foot resting on top of the weight-bearing foot.

IT band release with roller

Place a foam roller horizontally against a wall, just below your hip height. Stand side-on to a wall and rest the outside of your upper leg against the roller. Lean onto the roller with just enough weight that you can feel a gentle pressure but no pain.

Wait until you feel your leg softening, then shift the roller down your leg to the next tight point and repeat. This can be done all the way down to your knee. You can also start at your knee and work up if you find that way around works better for you. Check your other leg too, as the IT band is usually tight on both sides.

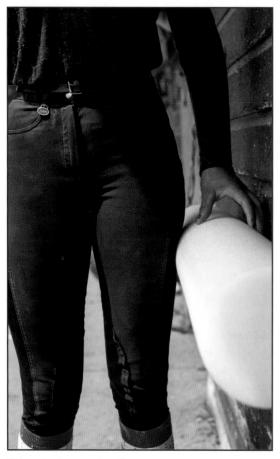

IT band release with roller.

Alternative releases:

* Chapter 5: Knee pain
* Chapter 6: Lower back too arched

■ PLANTAR FASCIITIS

The plantar fascia is the strong membrane on the sole of your foot that holds everything in its place. Plantar fasciitis is inflammation of this membrane.

The main symptom is pain, either in the heel or spreading under the foot or up into the Achilles tendon. The pain is particularly bad when you put weight on your foot first thing in the morning or after sitting for a time. In relatively mild cases, the pain wears off once you have started walking. My patients often describe having to hobble to the bathroom in the middle of the night or in the morning, but being able to walk normally after that.

Some people also develop bone spurs on their heel, which are small extra growths of bone that gradually develop in response to the irritation caused by chronic inflammation in the plantar fascia. While they are not themselves painful, they do cause pain in the surrounding tissues.

In my experience, the inflammation that starts this condition is caused by tightness in the muscles attaching into the sole of your foot, which is linked to tightness in the muscles in your upper leg, which tense up because the bones of your pelvis are rotated. I have successfully treated many people with plantar fasciitis without ever touching their feet. If you find and treat the cause of the problem, your body is normally able to heal the area of pain by completing the inflammatory cycle. For more information about this, see chapter 4.

How your riding is affected

Riding with your heels down can be tender if you have plantar fasciitis and difficult if your calves are tight. But this is actually a good position to be in for your feet, and will help to stretch your lower legs. Probably the most painful part for you will be dismounting and having to put weight through your heels again.

How to help yourself

Foot release with ball

Sit with the sole of your affected foot resting on a small ball. Some people use golf balls or spiky Pilates balls, which are fine if they work for you, but please go gently as too much pressure can cause bruising.

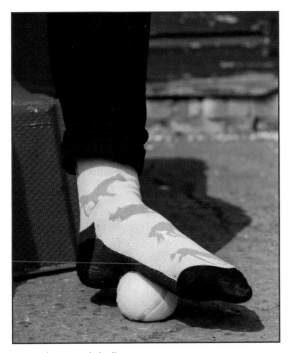

Foot release with ball.

Slowly roll your foot over the ball for a couple of minutes. If you find a spot that is very tight, just rest in that position until you feel it change and release. If any points are too painful to apply pressure into, then don't—you will still be helping those areas if you work around them.

Treat yourself

Sit with your affected foot on the floor and your knee bent at right angles. Place your other foot on the top of the affected foot in whatever position feels right.

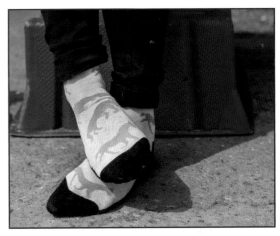

Treat yourself.

Apply gentle pressure from your top foot and hold for at least five minutes. If you feel that you need extra pressure, you can also push down through knee of the affected foot. But remember that you are not looking for pain, just your barrier. Then wait and sink down as your foot opens up. Stop if you have any increase in pain.

Finding a therapist who can assess and correct your pelvic alignment may be needed before these exercises are fully effective.

Alternative release:

♦ Chapter 6: Heels up

■ SCAR TISSUE

A scar is your body's way of replacing tissue that has been removed or damaged. It does this by laying down extra collagen fibers in the area as part of the healing process. This is an essential reaction, but scars can cause long-term problems for some people.

The scar that you get on your skin from an injury or operation is very obvious and you will be very aware of it if it is too tight or not healing properly. What is not so easy to detect is the internal scarring that occurs wherever tissue has been changed or disturbed. Sometimes, particularly after abdominal surgery, adhesions can form. These are bands of scar tissue that form between the scar tissue and organs, which can result in chronic pain and problems such as infertility. They can lead to ongoing symptoms that are not seen as coming directly from the injury. When excessive scarring occurs following joint surgery, it will cause pain and stiffness long after the expected recovery time.

Scars can remain tender both on the surface of the skin and in the tissues beneath for many years after they were formed. This is because of the nerve endings that become trapped and irritated by the restrictions in the fibers. They can also lead to chronic inflammation—I have seen many patients who have swelling in an area long after the initial injury has healed.

How your riding is affected

Any deep scars will alter your posture, strength, and flexibility in the local area, but they also have the potential to do the same in other areas of your body. This may be a subtle pull that you are not aware of, but your horse will almost certainly feel the effects that it has on your riding position. The illustration of fascia man on horse in chapter 2 clearly shows this effect.

How to help yourself

There are many products on the market that claim to reduce visible scarring; my opinion is that the more natural the product, the more likely it is to be able to work with your body to result in changes.

Internal scarring is more problematic, but if you are aware of the potential for postoperative problems then they are less likely to occur. Your surgeon will be able to tell you what the risks are and what can be done to minimize them if you discuss it before the operation. After the operation you can help yourself by doing the prescribed exercises, drinking plenty of water, and trying to move as normally as possible.

It is hard to give you specific advice on how to help problems caused by scars, as they are so individual. But in my experience, it is often possible to reduce their effects and the ongoing symptoms that they are causing. So if you are suffering, please find a practitioner who is trained in gentle scar release to find out if you can be helped.

If you are able to have gentle bodywork such as Myofascial Release, it will safely encourage the scar tissue fibers to lay down in the right direction, which makes the scar less likely to cause problems in the future. No treatment can eliminate scars, but their effects can be altered.

Treat yourself

Place your hand on the skin over your scar, allowing the weight of your hand to rest down and wait. Over a few minutes, the warmth and pressure from your hand will start to release the tissues in and around the scar—chapter 9 has all the details of how this works. You will probably find that the skin around your scar goes soft much more quickly, but just be patient and give the scar time to change—this will need regular treatments. If you are seeing a therapist, ask if there is anything specific you can do to help your scar, as I can only give very general advice here. As always, stop straight away if it is making any symptoms worse.

■ REPETITIVE STRAIN INJURY

According to the NHS website, "Repetitive strain injury (RSI) is a general term used to describe the pain felt in muscles, nerves and tendons caused by repetitive movement and overuse."[7]

It mainly affects your neck, shoulders, and arms and can produce symptoms such as pain, stiffness, swelling, numbness, tingling, and weakness. It is caused by activities that are repetitive, high intensity over a long period, or in an awkward position, forcing you into a poor posture. It is also known to get worse with vibrations, in the cold, or if you are stressed.

How your riding is affected

These symptoms can be aggravated by the repetitive motion of riding and having to sit and move in a certain way, which lead to other areas of your body tightening up in compensation.

How to help yourself

Identify the trigger

This is the most important thing that you can do for your RSI, remembering that there may be more than one trigger. If the cause is work related, your employer has a duty to provide you with the correct equipment and work conditions to prevent incidents of RSI where reasonably

possible. Making changes to the things that you spend all day doing will take the strain off your body and help it to heal the inflammation that has built up.

Working with horses can cause RSI too. So it is really important to use the right tools for the job, take breaks when you need to, and to vary your tasks throughout the day. There is a lot more information about how to do this in chapter 7.

There are suggestions of how you can treat specific joints further on in this chapter and in chapters 6 and 7.

■ HYPERMOBILITY

People with hypermobility syndrome have the ability to move their joints beyond the normal range—for example, being able to bend their thumbs back on themselves. It is sometimes known as being double jointed. This trait is often passed down through families and there are different grades of severity.

Some families are identified as having a particular syndrome such as Ehlers-Danlos syndrome (EDS), but many people do not realize that they are hypermobile until they have a problem. However, you can be hypermobile without having a serious condition. If you think that you may be hypermobile and are concerned about it, speak to your doctor, who will be able to run some tests and advise you on any treatment that you may need.

The hypermobility is caused by faulty collagen in your connective tissue fibers, which leads to looseness in structures throughout your body, such as ligaments and skin. The pain around joints that is a typical symptom is caused by recurrent soft-tissue damage from repeated overstretching.

How your riding is affected

For riders, this condition can be very painful, especially if you have a severe type of hypermobility disorder. But if you are aware of the potential problems and you manage your condition properly in your day-to-day activities, it is possible to continue riding.

Some of the most damaging movements for riders are those unexpected pulls and tugs from your horse, either when leading or riding. That is when you are unable to prepare yourself for the movement, so overstretching of joints is much more likely to happen.

How to help yourself

Find a therapist

Core-strengthening and joint-stabilizing exercises are the key to riding safely if you are hypermobile. I am not going to give any specific exercises or releases here, as there are too many variables in the condition and therefore you need to be assessed in person by someone who is qualified to advise you. This may be a therapist with training in exercise prescription, or someone such as a Pilates or yoga instructor who has experience in working with hypermobile people.

The releases that are shown in other sections of this book are very general and would normally be safe to do even with hypermobility. However, I would strongly encourage you to seek individual advice, maybe showing your therapist or exercise instructor this book, before you start anything new.

■ INCONTINENCE

The NHS estimates that three to six million people in the UK are living with urinary incontinence.[8]

In the US, over twenty-five million people have been diagnosed with urinary incontinence.[9]

Your pelvic floor is a sling of muscles that attaches to the bottom of your pelvis, supporting your pelvic organs and giving you control over your bladder and bowels. It is as important for men as for women, but often it is only mentioned or thought about after childbirth.

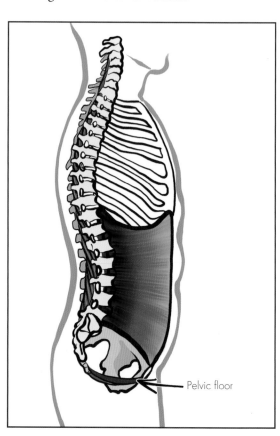

Pelvic floor

Urinary incontinence is normally blamed on a weak pelvic floor and sufferers are given exercises to strengthen it. This approach would be effective if that was the only reason, but remember that your pelvic floor is connected to the rest of your body, and it doesn't work in isolation. So if you have a history that includes back pain, pelvic rotation, childbirth, surgery or trauma (particularly in the abdominal or pelvic area), or pelvic organ prolapse, it is highly likely that they are contributing to the weakness.

Finding and treating the cause will be much more successful than doing exercises alone to try to overcome the problem. Once your pelvic floor is no longer tight and twisted because of strain from other areas of your body, the exercises will be much more effective.

How your riding is affected

Like your core muscles, the pelvic floor is used when you are riding for balance and to give you a soft seat, without you needing to particularly think about it. Regular horse riders tend to have a strong pelvic floor, but of course they can still be affected by same problems as nonriders.

There are two main types of urinary incontinence—stress and urge—with some people suffering from both. The causes and treatment are the same for each type in most cases, and men can be affected as well as women.

Stress incontinence is when the pelvic floor is unable to prevent urine from leaking when it is put under pressure. This may be when you cough, sneeze, or exercise. Riders tend to worry particularly when cantering or in sitting trot, although it will affect everyone slightly differently.

Urge incontinence is the inability to stop urine flow when your bladder feels that it is full, sometimes called an overactive bladder. It is why some people will always go to the bathroom "just in case" and will normally be very aware of when the next opportunity to go will be. For riders, going on long trail rides or to big events will be very problematic.

How to help yourself

Tell your doctor

So many people are embarrassed by this problem that they don't talk about it to their doctor or even friends and family. This has created a taboo that perpetuates the problem. In the first instance it is important for your doctor to rule out any conditions that may need medical intervention. Generally, the sooner problems are investigated and treated, the quicker and more successful the treatment.

There is worldwide controversy at the moment surrounding the use of vaginal mesh implants to treat incontinence. There are many women who have reported ill effects from the plastic polypropylene that is used, and as I write there are law suits in progress. This is a rapidly changing area as the investigations progress, so I would advise you to look into the most recent developments for yourself if you are considering this operation.

Get treatment

Find a therapist who is qualified in treating incontinence by looking at your whole body and finding the cause. The therapist will then be able to advise you on when and how to do the pelvic floor exercises. Ideally see someone who is qualified in assessing and treating your pelvic alignment; if the bones of your pelvis that the pelvic floor muscles are attached to are rotated, then it follows that your pelvic floor will also be twisted. For more information about your pelvic alignment, see chapter 1.

Pelvic floor exercises

Most women who have had children will have heard of Kegel exercises, but they apply to men too. These pelvic floor exercises were devised in the 1940s by Dr. Arnold Kegel, an American gynecologist.

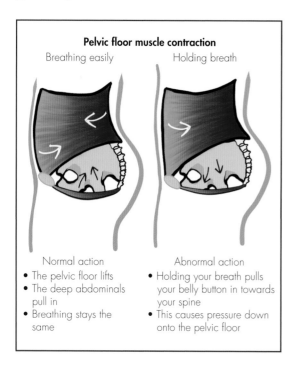

Pelvic floor muscle contraction

Breathing easily | Holding breath

Normal action
- The pelvic floor lifts
- The deep abdominals pull in
- Breathing stays the same

Abnormal action
- Holding your breath pulls your belly button in towards your spine
- This causes pressure down onto the pelvic floor

Begin with an empty bladder and slowly contract your pelvic floor from the back to the front of your body, as if you are trying to stop yourself from passing urine. Then hold the contraction for a count of ten (you might need to build up to

being able to maintain the contraction for that long) and slowly release the muscles until they are fully relaxed. Keep your breathing slow and gentle so that you do not hold your breath. But do not perform this exercise while you are passing urine as it can lead to incomplete bladder emptying and an increased risk of urinary infection.

Keep drinking

Although it may seem counterintuitive, it is very important to drink plenty of water to keep your bladder healthy. Limiting your fluid intake will increase the risk of infection and of bladder irritability. Sipping water throughout the day is a better way of keeping your body hydrated than gulping down lots in one go, and is less likely to put strain on your bladder if it is weak.

▪ REFERENCES

1. K. R. Meltzer, T. V. Cao, J. F. Schad, H. King, S. T. Stoll, and P. R. Standley. "In Vitro Modeling of Repetitive Motion Injury and Myofascial Release." *Journal of Bodywork and Movement Therapies* 14, no. 2 (2010): 162–71.

2. C. Greenough. "The National Back Pain Pathway." NHS England. Last modified 1 August 2016. https://www.england.nhs.uk/blog/charles-greenough/.

3. R. A. Deyo and Y. J. Tsui-Wu. "Descriptive Epidemiology of Low Back Pain and its Related Medical Care in the United States." *Spine* 12 (1987): 264–68.

4. N. E. Foster, J. R. Anema, D. Cherkin, R. Chou, S. P. Cohen, D. P. Gross, P. H. Ferreira, et al. "Prevention and Treatment of Low Back Pain: Evidence, Challenges, and

Promising Directions." *Lancet* 391, no. 10137 (2018): 2368–83.

5. S. Quinn and S. Bird. "Influence of Saddle Type upon the Incidence of Lower Back Pain in Equestrian Riders." *British Journal of Sports Medicine* 30, no. 2 (1996): 140–44.

6. G. Liptan, S. Mist, C. Wright, A. Arzt, and K. D. Jones. "A Pilot Study of Myofascial Release Therapy Compared to Swedish Massage in Fibromyalgia." *Journal of Bodywork and Movement Therapies* 17, no. 3 (2013): 365–70.

7. NHS UK. "Repetitive Strain Injury (RSI)." NHS Choices. Last modified 27 January 2016. https://www.nhs.uk/conditions/repetitive-strain-injury-rsi/.

8. D. E. Irwin, I. Milsom, Z. Kopp, P. Abrams, and L. Cardozo. "Impact of Overactive Bladder Symptoms on Employment, Social Interactions and Emotional Wellbeing in Six European Countries." *British Journal of Urology International* 97 (2005): 96–100.

9. National Association for Continence (NAFC). "Let's Get Past the Embarrassment and Get On with Our Lives." NAFC homepage. N.d., accessed 16 June 2018. https://www.nafc.org/home.

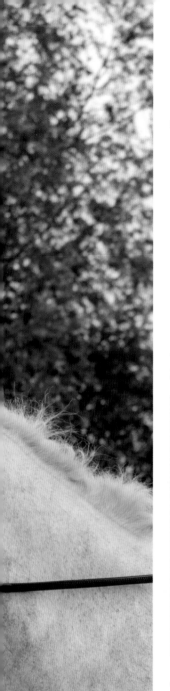

Solve Your Riding Problems the Myofascial Way

Please remember that the advice given in this chapter is general in nature and if you require individual advice, you should consult your own therapist.

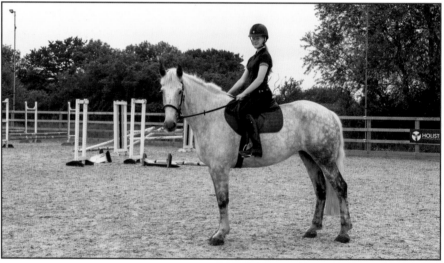

This chapter is not to going to teach you how to ride, but will show you a different way of approaching your riding issues.

How many times have you been told to correct the same thing by your riding instructor? Have you noticed that you always lean to the same side in photos of you riding? Are you tired of trying to force your body to do the right thing over and over again, only to feel that you are fighting it the whole time?

When you are learning to ride, as in any new exercise or skill, of course you need instruction and you will feel muscles that you didn't know existed working in ways that you had never imagined. But most of us, by the time we have learnt the basics, have also developed a range of new holding patterns and quirky movements. This is your body's way of compensating for old restrictions while still allowing you to do new things.

There is always a reason for problems, and remember that the cause may be in a different part of your body to the symptom. The following examples are only a small selection of the numerous ways in which your body can try to evade balance and symmetry. The suggestions I make are focused on helping you to recognize and feel what is happening, rather than simply changing your position.

Using photographs and video footage can be very helpful in allowing you to see what is happening and also to track your progress as things start to improve. Please don't expect to be able to correct everything in one go. I have ordered the problems by starting at the head and working down through the body, so you can choose to start in the place that affects you the most.

Having noted where your issue is, the next step is to feel. This is surprisingly difficult when you have spent many years trying to ignore what your body is telling you so that it doesn't stop you from doing what you need to do. So whether you are lying, standing, sitting in a chair, or sitting on your horse, just take a moment to feel.

- ◆ Do you have pain anywhere?
- ◆ Where can you feel pockets or lines of tension?
- ◆ Is your weight going through both sides of your body evenly?
- ◆ How is your breathing?
- ◆ Are you bracing anywhere?

The body scan: this is one way of getting used to feeling your body. Imagine that a tiny version of you is inside your body and is able to travel anywhere without any effort. Starting with your toes, slowly move up your body, taking note of any areas that are tight or sore. You can pause in those places and then allow your breathing to slow down, softening the tension and experiencing any sensations. Repeating this exercise when you are relaxed and not rushed will gradually make it easier to feel what is happening in your body and it will become much more obvious to you when something is causing your body to react. If you can feel, then you will be able to do something about the problem by changing the cause of it, not just forcing against it.

All the exercises and stretches that I suggest in this chapter are very gentle and should always be performed in a slow, controlled way. But sometimes you may have symptoms that are a sign of a more serious problem, are related to something else going on in your body, or that are simply too irritable for the exercise that you are trying. So please make sure that you only do what you feel confident with and that you stop immediately if you are unsure, if anything that you are doing doesn't feel right, or if your symptoms begin to get worse. If this does happen it is best to get checked by a health professional or bodyworker before you do any more exercises. Remember that the advice given in this book is very general and cannot replace assessment and treatment from someone who can see and feel exactly what your specific problems are.

The exercises described in this section are focused on releases rather than strengthening, as the principles of Myofascial Release (the treatment technique that I specialize in) show that it is essential to achieve the correct starting position before attempting to strengthen any weakness. A lot of the time, apparent weaknesses occur simply because of tension in the opposing muscle group. I have treated athletes who go on to achieve personal bests in the days following their treatment. Their muscles cannot have become significantly bigger in that time, but when the tension is released from within and around a muscle, it is able to work much more efficiently straight away.

You may already know exercises or releases to help the problems that I describe here, and, of course, if they help you there is no reason to stop doing them. However, you may find that these alternative suggestions are more practical on the yard or that they are good to add into your repertoire.

Remember that it doesn't matter how far you move, just focus on what you feel. It is normal to move a different amount each time you do the same release, and the two sides of your body are likely to move in different ways too. If you know that you are a competitive person, try not to give yourself goals of how far you are going to go or how much you are going to do. This approach may be frustrating to begin with, but once you learn how to feel and follow your body, you will be able to work with it and not against it. Then your symptoms will become easier to manage and you will be able to prevent further problems in the future.

The contract/relax method: in some of the exercises I will talk about this technique, which will be used to help different areas of your body. This way of exercising is very effective in helping you to feel where existing tightness is held, and teaching your muscles the difference between tension and relaxation. As you have probably experienced, it is much easier to contract a tight muscle than to relax it when you try. So rather than advising you to relax the tight area, I will

show you how to tighten into it first, then hold for a count of ten, and very slowly and gently allow it to soften and let go until it is limp and relaxed. Remember not to push into pain, though.

A note about foam rollers: You may have seen people vigorously rolling up and down on their foam roller, probably grimacing and quite possibly groaning in pain while they do it. Please do not roll on your roller! Research has shown that the effects of rolling on joint mobility are limited to ten minutes,[1] and that it has the potential to cause tissue damage by the pressure that is exerted on the connective tissue, nerves, and blood vessels.[2]

The kinder and more effective way of using your foam roller is to lie or lean against it with the part of your body that you are trying to release. Then wait for at least five minutes to give your tissues a chance to change in response to the sustained pressure. If you do feel a release then it is fine to gently move into the next area of restriction that you feel, and then wait again. In this way, you will not hurt yourself as you are always following what you feel and not forcing any changes on your body.

POSTURE

In this section I have picked out some common postural problems when you are riding, but if they are present in the saddle, the chances are they are also going to be affecting other activities in your life. Then, in the next chapter, I will talk you through how to help your posture when you are working on the yard.

What about your life away from horses, though? In chapter 8 I will talk about some of the other factors that can affect your posture. You may even find that changing something that you do at home or work will improve your riding.

■ CHIN FORWARD

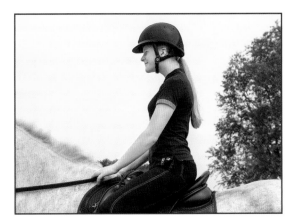

Chin-forward posture.

This posture is due to tightness in your jaw, throat, and upper chest pulling your head too far in front of your neck. The exercises that are usually given to correct this are to strengthen the muscles in the back of your neck to pull your head back into the correct position. But if you are still holding on to a lot of tension at the front, this will be very difficult and is likely to create a tug-of-war between the muscles at the front and the back of your neck.

How your riding is affected

Your head is relatively heavy (on average 10 lb or 5 kg) so having a chin-forward posture pulls down on your neck and shoulders. This in turn will make you slouch and change how you are sitting in the saddle.

How to help yourself

Treat yourself

Place one hand skin on skin onto your sternum (breast bone) and allow the weight of your arm

to gently hang down, without moving your hand over the top of the skin.

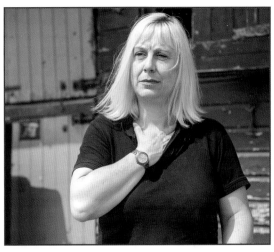

Treat yourself.

Allow your hand to sink in and follow any movements that you feel under your hand. Don't worry if you don't feel much, you will still be helping yourself by staying with it. If your head begins to move as you release that is fine, but don't try to move it consciously. When you have finished, keep your hand in the same place until you have lifted your arm slightly, then very slowly peel your hand away. This can be done sitting or standing. Remember to breathe and aim to hold for a minimum of five minutes.

Alternative release:

◆   Chapter 5: Neck pain

■ HEAD TILTED TO ONE SIDE

This may be as simple as being in the habit of looking down at your horse's shoulder when you are riding—for example, checking if you are on the correct diagonal in trot or on the correct leg in canter.

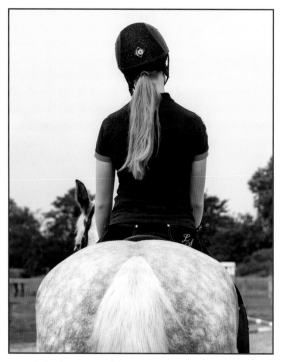

Head tilted to one side.

However, this posture could also be due to several different conditions and if you have extreme pain or if you are unable to straighten your head when you try to, it is very important to seek medical attention before attempting any self-treatment.

One reason is torticollis or wry neck, which is a very painful condition caused by tightness or spasm of the muscles in one side of your neck. It can appear to come on suddenly and for no apparent reason, but is normally linked to asymmetry and tightness elsewhere in your body. This will probably respond well to hands-on treatment, but you can treat yourself too.

If you have been told that your head tilts to one side but you were not aware of it, it is possibly related to previous traumas such as head injury, concussion, or whiplash. These events may have resulted in tightness in one side of your neck or even a balance problem relating to your inner ear. When the signals going to your brain are distorted, over time it reduces your brain's ability to react to the forces of gravity and so your head-tilted posture feels normal to you. This can result in symptoms such as headaches, jaw and facial pain, and vertigo. If you are experiencing any of these symptoms following a trauma and you have not been checked by a medical professional, please do get seen to make sure that you do not have any injuries that need treatment.

How your riding is affected

The more you can feel what your body is doing when you are riding, the less time you will need to spend looking down. So, using video and feedback from your instructor will be very helpful to break the habit of having to look down.

The side to which your head is tilted tends to get tension into the shoulder, arm, and hand. This reduces the sensitivity and effectiveness of your hand, resulting in problems with resistance in the horse's mouth. The head tilt will also pull your whole body toward that side, shifting your weight and making your horse have to compensate.

How to help yourself

Use heat

This is really effective in helping to relax tight painful muscles, so having a warm bath or shower is a good starting point. Using a hot pack that you can mold to the shape of your neck is also very soothing.

Treat yourself

This is the same as with the elevated shoulders section in this chapter, but place your hand wherever you are tightest. This may change each time you treat yourself, so it is worth taking your time to feel where you need to treat.

Alternative release:

+ Chapter 6: Shoulders elevated

■ ROUNDED SHOULDERS

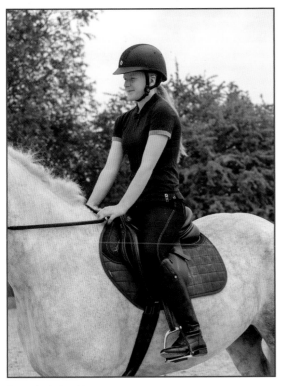

Rounded shoulders.

If your shoulders are normally held forward and you feel that you constantly have to brace them back to correct them, then they are not going to be any different when you are riding. This is a very common problem and people are often advised to strengthen their back muscles to pull the shoulders back to correct them. But, if you think about it, your shoulders are being pulled forward from the front of your body—it is the tightness at the front that causes the problem, not weakness at the back.

The main muscles that tend to be too tight are the pectorals, which attach in a fan shape from the top of your humerus just below your shoulder, under the clavicle (collar bone), and into the side of the sternum (breast bone). When the pectoral muscles are pulling your shoulders forward, it puts a lot of strain on your upper back, which then has to work harder to keep you upright. So you will often get pain and burning between your shoulder blades if your shoulders are rounded.

How your riding is affected

Rounded shoulders will alter your balance and reduce your upper-body control. Then, other areas of your body will need to tense up to maintain your balance when riding, which shifts your weight distribution in the saddle. A common result of poor balance is tensing up into your arms and hands, which will pull into your horse's mouth.

How to help yourself

Shoulder stretch with upright post

This is a great release that can be done anywhere that has an upright post to lean on. Door frames are also good for this. Remember, never force or move into pain, just feel for your comfortable end point and wait there until it softens. This release should be done on both sides of your body, and if one side is worse than the other, do the best side first. This is to make things easier for your body to change, and by releasing the looser side you will start to open up the tighter side before you get there.

Stand by the post with the side you are working on closest to it. With your elbow bent and relaxed, place the palm of your hand, facing forward, flat onto the post.

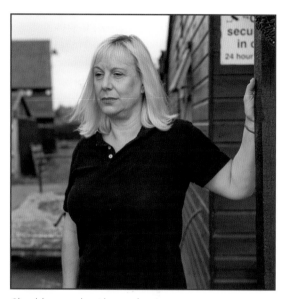

Shoulder stretch with upright post.

Slowly turn away from the post until you feel a gentle pull in the front of your shoulder and into your chest. Then wait at that point until you feel that the pull has lessened or that you are able to move further into the stretch with your body. You can then slowly bring your body back to the center and relax your arm, or wait at the next pull that you feel, and repeat.

Alternative release:

◆   Chapter 5: Neck pain

■ SHOULDERS ELEVATED

This is when your shoulders are held up toward your ears, often without you realizing until you spot yourself in a mirror or someone else points it out to you. Holding your shoulders in this way

may be associated with stress, or it may simply have become a habit that feels normal.

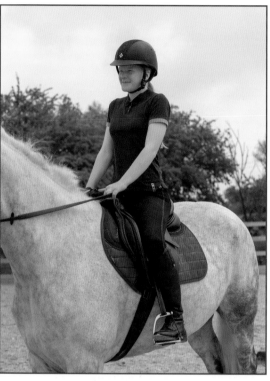

Shoulders elevated.

When you are feeling stressed, your shoulders tend to creep up, which increases the tension in your muscles, causing pain, increasing stress, and so on until it becomes a vicious circle. The trouble is, once this becomes your normal position, your brain gets desensitized to it and it is harder to pick up on when it is happening.

Some people spend their lives with their shoulders up around their ears, and others get the shoulder creep when they do certain things. If you are cold, nervous, or stressed when you are riding, it is more likely to happen.

The main muscle causing your shoulders to rise up is called the upper trapezius. This muscle is the upper part of the larger trapezius muscle, and is the hard, knotted area between your neck and the top of your shoulder.

How your riding is affected

This is a position of tension that your horse will pick up on very quickly, reducing the communication between you and making it harder for you and your horse to be sensitive to each other's needs.

How to help yourself

Treat yourself

Place your hand skin on the skin over the top of your opposite upper trapezius (between your neck and shoulder), and allow gravity to take the weight of your arm.

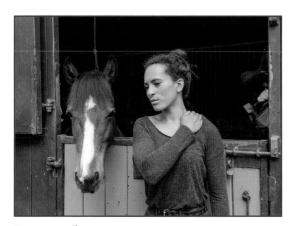

Treat yourself.

Without moving your hand over the top of your skin, allow your hand to sink in until you feel a release. When you have finished, keep your hand in the same place until you have lifted your arm slightly, then very slowly peel your hand away. Repeat on the opposite side (start with your best side). This can be done sitting or standing.

Remember to breathe and aim to hold for a minimum of five minutes.

Alternative release:

◆ Chapter 6: Holding your breath

■ ONE SHOULDER FURTHER FORWARD

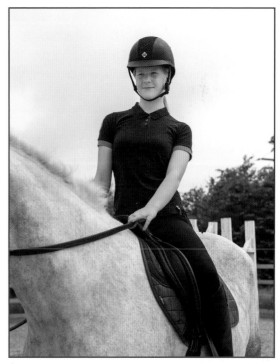

One shoulder further forward.

This posture can have several different causes, so it would be worth trying a few approaches to find the one that helps you the most. Don't forget to check your pelvic alignment, as if your pelvis is rotated it will tend to pull one side of your body further forward.

If one of your pectoral muscles is tighter than the other, it can pull the shoulder on that side further forward: see the release under the rounded shoulders section. Or it could be due to tightness in your scapula (shoulder blade) on the opposite side. If the muscle tension is pulling your shoulder blade back, it will look as though your opposite shoulder is too far forward.

How your riding is affected

The shoulder that is being held further back will develop more tension, which will cause a twist through your trunk. So, to maintain your balance you will need to grip the rein tighter on that side. Then your horse is subjected to the forces from your twists both from the saddle and through the reins into its mouth.

How to help yourself

The post lean

This is good for releasing around your shoulder blade. It can be done with the corner of a wall or post, and I also find that door frames work well for me.

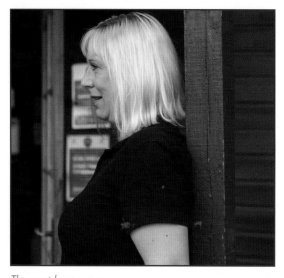

The post lean.

Stand with the inside of your shoulder blade against the corner of the upright post and gently lean into it, using your body weight, not force. Stop before it is painful, waiting wherever you feel resistance. As your tension starts to release, slowly allow yourself to sink further onto the corner. Wait until you feel that the shoulder on that side is able to fall forward slightly or that the arm drops.

Alternative release:

♦   Chapter 6: Rounded shoulders

■ ONE SHOULDER LOWER

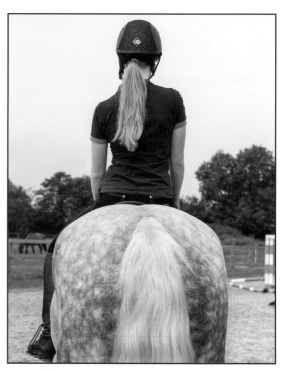

One shoulder lower.

This may actually be because your opposite shoulder is being pulled up by the upper trapezius muscle. Or your shoulder might be pulled lower by tension in your waist on that side. There are several muscles that could contribute to this and, as they tend to work together, you do not need to know exactly which ones are to blame.

How your riding is affected

This posture will again produce tension through your hands into your horse's mouth in an asymmetrical way. Over time this will result in tension in your horse's neck too.

How to help yourself

Side stretch

Find a surface that is about waist height, such as the top of a stable half door, the back of a chair, or a worktop. Stand sideways with your highest shoulder toward it, and lean sideways over the surface.

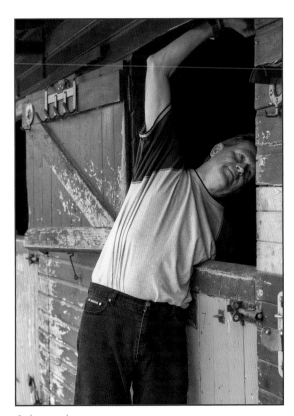

Side stretch.

Only go as far as is comfortable, using your arms to support you if needed. Then rest in that position until you feel your body softening and you are able to slowly move further into the stretch. When you have finished come up gradually, using your arms to help you up. The back of a heavy chair can also be good for this. Remember to keep breathing.

Alternative release:

* Chapter 6: Shoulders elevated

■ ELBOWS HELD OUT

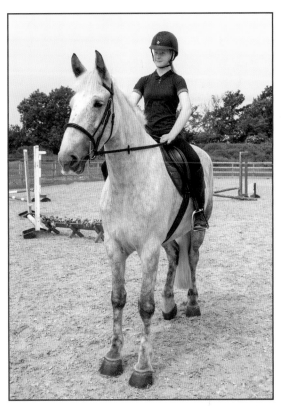

Elbows held out.

If you find it difficult to keep your elbows tucked into your sides, you probably have tightness in the muscles that rotate your shoulders inward. If you have a history of trauma to the area, it might also be linked to weakness in the opposite muscle groups that should stabilize your shoulder position. Check whether you are holding your elbows too far forward too, as this will change the angle.

How your riding is affected

Tension in your shoulders and arms makes it much harder to ride with soft hands, increasing the pull into your horse's mouth through the reins.

How to help yourself

Shoulder rotators release

Stand in a doorway or against a post with your elbow bent, and rest the inside of your forearm against the post. Relax your shoulders and remember to breathe. Keeping your arm in that position, slowly turn your body away from the post until you feel a resistance, but no pain.

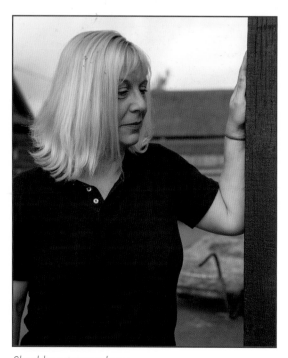

Shoulder rotators release.

Hold at that point until you feel the tightness start to soften. Then you can either follow it to the next point of resistance and repeat, or slowly bring your body back to the center and take the stretch off your arm.

Alternative release:

- Chapter 6: Rounded shoulders

■ GRIPPING YOUR REINS TOO HARD

This problem is probably linked to tension in your arms and upper body, but there are several possible reasons for it. A tight grip could be a sign of anxiety, reacting to either the horse that you are riding or the situation. It may also be in compensation for lack of balance elsewhere in your body, meaning that you have to hold on tighter to maintain your balance.

How your riding is affected

Whether or not your tight grip is as a result of your stress or anxiety, your horse will probably interpret it that way, and it may then become "fizzed up" and not listen to you. The tight grip will also reduce your sensitivity and contact through the reins.

How to help yourself

Contract/relax for arms

This exercise is good for tension in your arms as well as in your hands. Even if you think that only one side is tight, it is better to do this exercise with both arms at the same time, helping symmetry in your body and releasing tension that you might not realize is there.

Starting with your hands, slowly make a fist. Then spread that tension up through your wrists, elbows, and shoulders, curling your arms up as tightly as you can.

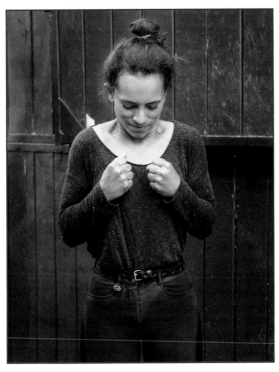

Contract/relax for arms.

Hold for a count of ten and then very slowly release and soften both arms and hands until they are completely limp. Repeat three times.

Alternative release:

◆　Chapter 5: Hand and wrist pain and stiffness

■ HOLDING YOUR BREATH

This is a really common thing that lots of people do in their everyday lives without ever realizing it. If it is a habit that you have got into, you probably do it when you are riding too. It can be caused by tension in your upper body, bracing yourself ready for a problem, or a tight diaphragm. For more information about breathing and how to use your diaphragm, have a look at chapter 8.

How your riding is affected

If your horse is sensitive, it may interpret your breath holding as tension, and also tense itself up. When you are holding your breath it is hard to keep your hands soft, and so your horse will also feel it into its mouth.

How to help yourself

Diaphragm release

Stand with a roller or half roller across the middle of your back and lean onto it against a wall. Just rest there, using the weight of your body to allow your tissues to melt around the roller, until you feel a softening.

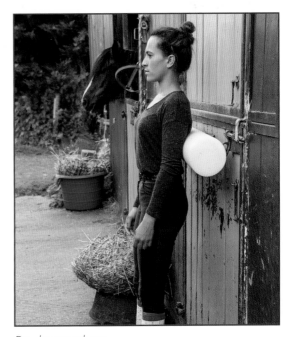

Diaphragm release.

To increase the intensity, try raising your arms above your head. But remember that you are feeling for resistance, not pain. Aim to hold for at least five minutes. This can also be done lying on your back with the foam roller on the floor or bed, or sitting with the roller against the back of the chair.

Alternative releases:

- Chapter 7: At the end of the day
- Chapter 8: Breathe properly

■ SITTING WITH MORE WEIGHT THROUGH ONE BUTTOCK

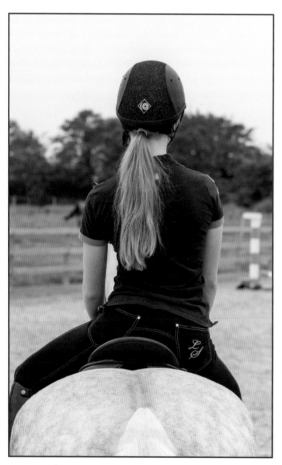

Sitting with more weight through one buttock.

Assuming that you are not being thrown out of balance by an imbalance in your horse or saddle, this postural problem is probably linked to your pelvic or spinal alignment. If your pelvis is rotated or you have a twist or curve in your spine, it will make it almost impossible for you to sit with your weight evenly distributed on both sides. In fact, trying to correct it by changing the way that you sit when you are riding is very likely to lead to tension and pain in other areas of your body that then have to work harder in compensation.

How your riding is affected

If your spine is curved or twisted, your whole body will also be pulled with it, causing your horse to have to compensate massively. If your weight is guiding your horse toward a direction different from where you think you should be heading, you and your horse will be trying to move in different directions. This will obviously reduce your ability to work with your horse and will affect you in all paces.

How to help yourself

Check your saddle

Has it worn unevenly or is there damage causing asymmetry? If you share your tack with another rider or you bought it second-hand, this problem may have been caused by someone else's poor posture as well as your own. If you can see uneven wear, a saddle fitter will be able to easily give you advice and correct it.

Check your horse

As I talked about in chapter 1, you and your horse will affect each other's position and can cause problems for each other. So, if you are having postural issues, it is worth getting your horse's pelvis and back assessed and treated if necessary.

Check your body

Find a bodyworker who is qualified to look at the position of your spine to check if your pelvis is rotated. Try to get this treated and corrected as soon as possible to prevent issues developing in the rest of your body. Remember that if you have been riding the same horse with those twists in your body, the horse may also be compensating for them.

■ LOWER BACK TOO ARCHED

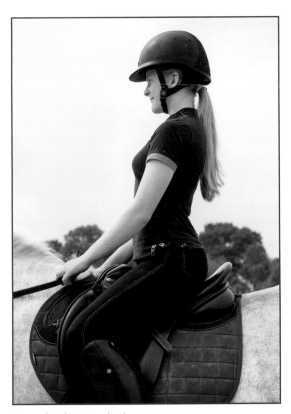

Lower back too arched.

If your pelvis is tilting forward when you are riding, causing your back to arch too much, it is probably always held like that, even if you are not aware of it. Tightness in your psoas and quadriceps (thigh) muscles on both sides will arch your back in this way.

How your riding is affected

This posture is sometimes connected with you trying to urge the horse forward more, as well as the position of your pelvis. It will alter the way that your weight is transmitted through your pelvis and into the stirrups, changing your leg position. Then the balance of both you and your horse will be compromised.

How to help yourself

Psoas release with chair

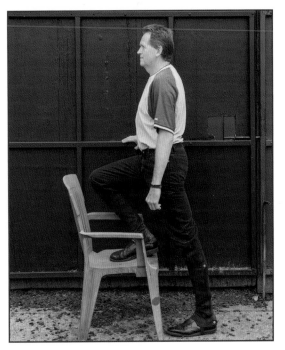

Psoas release with chair.

Put one foot up in front of you onto a surface approximately 30"/76 cm high, such as a chair or mounting block. Lean forward until you have flexed your hip and leg as far as possible. Then, holding at that point, lean your trunk backward, stretching the front of your opposite hip and thigh.

Hold in a gentle but sustained stretch for four to five minutes, or long as you are comfortable. Repeat on the opposite side. If necessary, you can use a lower surface, but you might need to stand farther away in order for the stretch to be effective. It is fine to steady yourself with one hand while doing this release.

Thigh release with chair

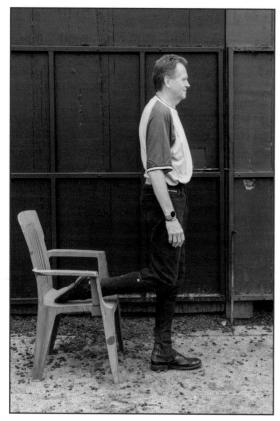

Thigh release with chair.

For this exercise you can use a chair, mounting block, or low wall. Stand with your back to the chair, holding on to the back of the chair or a wall if you need to keep your balance. Standing on one leg, bend the knee of your other leg and rest the top of your foot on the chair for support. Keep your knees together, and elongate your bent knee toward the floor.

Actively lift your hip on the side being released to level it with the other one. Wait until you feel the release in the front of your thigh, then slowly straighten your leg. Repeat with your other leg to help your pelvic area to stay symmetrical. Choose the chair height based your height and on the flexibility of your knee and thigh muscles, and hold on if you need to.

Alternative release:

- Chapter 5: Knee pain

■ LOWER BACK COLLAPSED

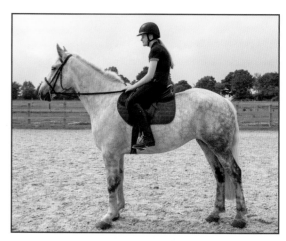

Lower back collapsed.

This is when your pelvis is tilted backward, which may be linked to weak core muscles and tension in your gluteal (buttock) muscles. As I have said previously, it is a good idea to release the tension in the tight muscles before trying to strengthen the weak ones.

It is very common in women returning to riding after having a baby, especially if they had a caesarean section. But any abdominal surgery, such as hysterectomy, will have the same effect.

How your riding is affected

If you are slumped in the saddle, you will tend to pull more on the reins, altering your balance and slowing your horse down.

How to help yourself

Buttock release with ball

You may find that there are some very tender areas deep in your buttocks, so start by sitting on the ball, placing the ball in an area that is tight but not too painful. Then wait until you can feel it start to soften and melt, then you can shift to move the ball to the next bit that needs releasing. Aim to do this release for at least five minutes.

■ TOES POINTING OUTWARD

This common problem is caused when tension, either in your hip or lower leg, is stronger on the outside than the inside, so it rotates your leg—and therefore your toes—outward. It will also occur if you have a weakness in your inner leg, resulting in an imbalance and your leg rotating outward. If you do need to strengthen some of your muscles, it is important first to release tightness in the area as you will otherwise be fighting to correct a problem that isn't the root

cause. You might find that this is an issue in only one of your legs, or both. Either way, it is a good idea to do the exercise with both legs.

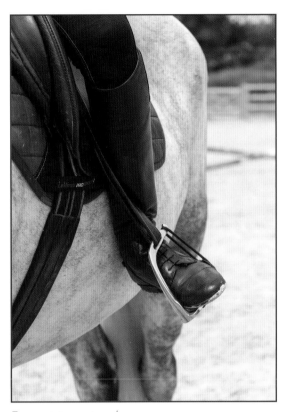

Toes pointing outwards.

How your riding is affected

If you are riding with your toes sticking out, it is harder to maintain contact with your horse's sides and so you are more likely to have to grip too hard with your upper legs.

How to help yourself

Contract/relax for lower legs

Start off sitting on a chair, and then progress this exercise to when you are mounted on your horse.

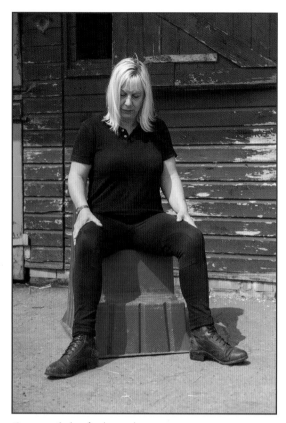

Contract/relax for lower legs.

Turn your legs outward, tightening into the tense bits as hard as you can, hold for a count of ten and then very slowly soften all your tension until your legs are feeling really limp and relaxed. Repeat three times. Do not move into pain.

Alternative release:

♦ Chapter 5: Hip pain, IT band

▦ HEELS UP

If you have tight calves and Achilles tendons, you will find it very difficult to ride with your heels well down. You may naturally have shortness in the tendons that attach your calf muscles to the bone, in which case both legs will be affected,

or it might have developed over time following injuries or bad habits—it is then more likely to be one-sided. Many women suffer from this if they wear (or used to wear) high heels.

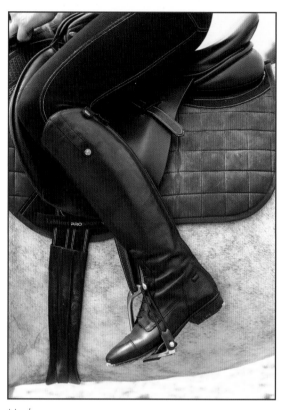

Heels up.

You also need to check the position of your lower legs. If they are too far back, your toes will be thrown forward and your heels will rise up. The opposite also applies.

How your riding is affected

Whether the cause of this posture is your leg position or shortening of your calf muscles, riding with your heels up makes it difficult to balance through your legs. So you will have to tense up your upper body and arms to compensate.

How to help yourself

Calf release with ball

Place a tennis ball between your calf muscle and a hard surface, positioning the ball in an area that you can feel is tight, but that is not too painful to put gentle pressure into.

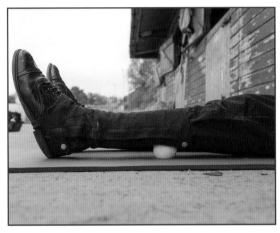

Calf release with ball.

This can be easily done while leaning against wall, but you can also use the ball in this way when you are sitting on the floor with your legs outstretched or lying on your back. If you feel that you need a bit more help to release the muscle, you can try moving your foot around any tight points that you come across.

Aim to stay resting with the ball in the same place until you can feel that the area has softened and started to release. Then you can allow the ball to roll until you find another area of restriction, and wait there for the release again. This stretch should take at least five minutes to be effective.

Alternative release:

◆   Chapter 5: Plantar fasciitis

■ GRIPPING TOO HARD WITH YOUR LEGS

As with many of these problems, the possible causes are very connected with each other. If you are feeling insecure when you are riding, it will make you tend to grip on, especially with your upper legs. But if you already have tightness in your hip adductors (the inner parts of your thighs) it makes it very hard to relax them and reduce the grip around your horse and relax your seat. So then a vicious cycle is set up and the problem gradually gets worse.

How your riding is affected

Gripping with your legs will pull your upper body forward and cause a change in balance for your whole body. As this in turn results in decreased control, you will probably need to grip even more tightly with your legs.

How to help yourself

Hip adductor stretch

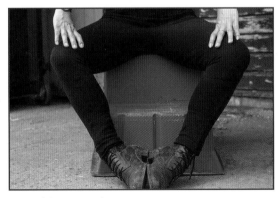

Hip adductor stretch.

Sit on a chair or mounting block. Turn your feet in so that the soles are touching each other in front of you on the ground (it is fine to do this with riding or yard boots on, but it might be more comfortable to take them off). Allow your knees to fall open away from each other, keeping your back and shoulders soft.

This release is about feeling for resistance on the inside of your thighs, but it should be passive, so you are not actively moving your legs apart. To find the point of resistance (but never pain), rest your hands on the inside of your legs and slowly open them. Stop in whatever position you start to feel a gentle tightness, and wait. This may be at a different angle for each leg, and will change each time that you do the release. Wait at your barrier until the insides of your thighs have softened and released, then allow them to open until you feel the next point of resistance, and repeat.

Alternative release:

* Chapter 6: Unable to swing your right leg over

MOUNTING AND DISMOUNTING

■ DIFFICULTY STEPPING UP WITH YOUR LEFT LEG

This could be because of arthritic changes in your left hip—see chapter 5 to find out more about arthritis. It could also be linked to tightness in your left buttock, or in both buttocks. Tension in the muscles at the front of your right hip (psoas and quadriceps) will pull you forward on the right, making it more difficult to balance and stretch forward with your left leg.

How to help yourself

Hip-loosening exercise

This will help to increase the range of motion of your left hip. Stand on your right leg with your hand touching something to help you balance. Starting with your left toes on the ground, slowly draw increasing circles with your left leg. As the circles get bigger, allow your foot to come up off the ground and bend your hip and knee more.

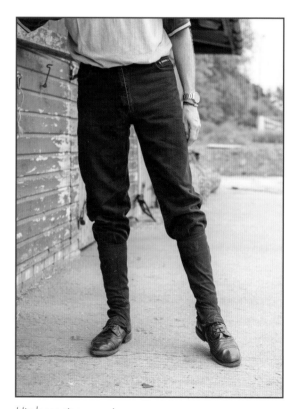

Hip-loosening exercise.

Keep going, gradually moving your hip more into the range of movement until you have your foot at the right height to reach the stirrups. It will probably take you a few weeks to improve this, so take your time and do not force into pain.

You can, of course, do the same exercise for your right hip if that is also stiff.

Alternative releases:

- Chapter 6: Lower back too arched
- Chapter 6: Unable to straighten up after you have dismounted
- Chapter 6: Knee pain during rising trot

■ UNABLE TO SWING RIGHT LEG OVER

As with gripping your legs too hard when you are riding, this problem is associated with tightness in your hip adductors or inner thighs. It could just be on one side but is usually in both legs to some degree, and tightness in either side will make it difficult to mount your horse.

How to help yourself

Contract/relax for hips

To start with, sit on a firm surface with both feet flat on the floor and slightly apart. Make fists with both hands and place them on the insides of your knees so they are touching each other. You could use a soccer ball instead if you find it easier.

Squeeze your knees in toward each other until you are using the muscles at about eighty percent of their maximum contraction, so that you are squashing your fists or the ball. Hold this contraction for a count of ten, then very slowly soften your legs and release the grip until both legs are fully relaxed. Repeat three times.

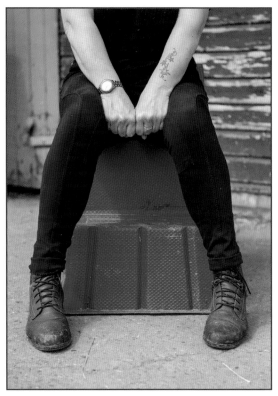

Contract/relax for hips.

Alternative release:

- Chapter 6: Gripping your legs too hard

■ UNABLE TO STRAIGHTEN UP AFTER DISMOUNTING

If you find yourself still bending over once your feet are back on the ground, your lower back is probably being pulled forward by tight psoas muscles. (For more information on what psoas is and how it works, see chapter 5.) This might be because they are always tight and probably causing lower back pain, or they might have reacted to something that happened when you were riding— for example, you were tensing up from trying something new, or having to sit a spook.

How to help yourself

Direct psoas release

This release is easy to do when you first dismount, and you can even still have the reins hanging off your arm as long as you have a docile horse that will patiently wait for you to straighten up.

Stand with equal weight through both legs and hook your thumbs in behind the bones at the front of your pelvis. It may feel very tight and tender there, so just sink in as far as you can comfortably go.

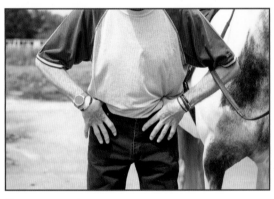

Direct psoas release.

Wait for the tightness to start releasing, which should be after about two minutes. This will happen gradually, allowing your bottom to tuck in and your back to straighten up. Don't worry if the two sides release at different times, just keep on the gentle pressure with both thumbs and wait for them to level up.

This is also good to do when you are still mounted if you feel that your back is beginning to seize up. If you are sitting it might be a bit harder to find the bones, but the technique is just the same as when you are standing. If you know that this tends to happen to you, practicing finding the right place when you are sitting in a chair might be helpful.

Alternative release:

♦   Chapter 6: Lower back too arched

■ REFERENCES

1.   C. Beardsley and J. Skarabot. "Effects of Self-Myofascial Release: A Systematic Review." *Journal of Bodywork and Movement Therapies* 19, no. 4 (2015): 747–58.
2.   P. F. Curran, R. D. Fiore, and J. J. Crisco. "A Comparison of the Pressure Exerted on Soft Tissue by 2 Myofascial Rollers." *Journal of Sport Rehabilitation* 17, no. 4 (2008): 432–42.

CHAPTER 7

On the Yard

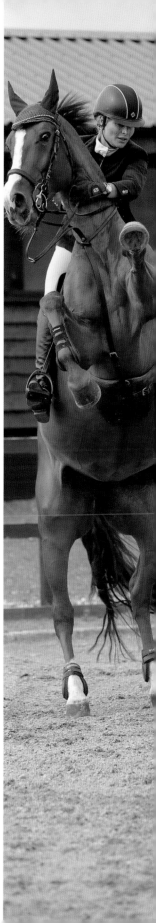

Please remember that the advice given in this chapter is general in nature and if you require individual advice, you should consult your own therapist.

The everyday jobs that need doing on every yard are so routine for most horse people, that you probably don't even remember the first time that you were shown what to do. In fact, were you ever actually shown how to do things properly? Or did you just pick it up by watching everyone else and learning from your own mistakes?

The problem comes when everyone accepts that they have to live with pain, and that they feel the need to push through and get everything done as quickly as possible. I expect that if I asked, you would be able to tell me how things should be done in an ideal world, given lots of time, space, and money. So, apologies if I tell you things that you already know—most of this chapter is common sense, but sometimes we need to be told things in a different way for them to make sense and to see how to apply them to our lives.

The aim of this chapter is to recognize that life isn't always ideal and to suggest ways of doing things that work for you in the real world. I would like to change the culture of the yard to one of taking care of yourself and doing the jobs safely. Working in a way that doesn't damage your body will allow you to keep riding for longer and more comfortably.

As with all the advice that I give in this book, it is very important to follow what you feel and to stop if what you are doing makes any symptoms worse or if it doesn't feel right. It could be that you need to receive a course of hands-on treatment to help existing conditions before you are able to follow these suggestions. That would be worth doing, as once you are balanced and not in pain all the time, it will be much easier to do things properly.

■ LIFTING

Learning how to lift and move heavy objects safely is essential when working with horses. Following this advice will not only help to prevent injuries, but will allow you to use your body in a kind way so that your muscles don't have to tighten up to protect themselves.

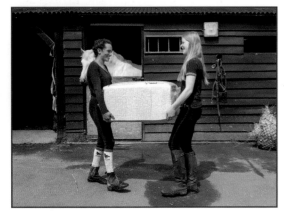

Lifting safely.

How to lift safely

1. **Think before you start to lift:** Take a minute to look at where you will be moving the load to—is there a clear path from where you will be starting, or are there obstructions? Will you need help either to lift it in the first place or once you get there? Is there a place to rest if you need to change your grip or if you are struggling?

2. **Hold the load close to your waist:** Keeping the load close to your waist will reduce the amount of pressure on your back. Hold the heaviest side next to your body and try to move it as close to you as possible before trying to lift it.

3. **Check that you have a stable position:** Your feet should be placed comfortably apart with one leg slightly further forward to help with your balance. Remember that you may need to shift the position of your feet during the lift to stay stable. If you are wearing unsuitable footwear it will make this much more difficult (yard or riding boots are perfect).

4. **Make sure you have a good grip on the load:** Depending on the size of the load relative to the length of your arms, you may need to make a few adjustments to your grip before you start the lift. If you do need to change your grip, put the load down first. This might be the time to ask for help if you can feel that your grip isn't firm enough.

5. **Do not bend your back when you are lifting:** Your spine should not be perfectly straight as it naturally curves slightly in at the bottom, out in the middle, and in again at your neck. But if you bend it forward to lift, it puts enormous pressure on your back and that is when injuries occur. So, at the start of the lift bend your knees and hips, sticking your bottom out if needed, to get down to the same level as the load.

6. **Keep your back in a good position while you are lifting:** Keep your hips and knees bent while you are starting to raise the load up, and bring it close into your body before straightening your legs again.

7. **Do not twist when you lift:** Avoid twisting your back or leaning sideways—keep your shoulders level and facing the same direction as your hips. When you change direction, step around so that your whole body follows your feet instead of turning your upper body.

8. **Look ahead of you:** Once you have lifted the load, try not to look down as this will start to bend your back. That is why checking that the path is clear before you start is a good idea.

9. **Move smoothly:** Keep your movements slow and controlled, so that you can feel

what the load and your body are doing. Then, if there is a problem you will have more chance of making adjustments to correct it or of putting the load down safely.

10. **Know your limits:** Just because you are able to lift something doesn't mean that you should lift it! The lifting that we are talking about here is part of the daily repetitive jobs that need doing, not just a one-off load. That makes a massive difference to the strain that is put on your body and is what is likely to lead to problems. So if you are in doubt, please get help.

11. **Don't bend your back when putting the load down:** Having lifted the load with a perfect posture, moved your feet and controlled your movements, please don't then hurt yourself by putting it down without thinking. You need to do the same bending of hips and knees, and sticking your bottom out, as when you lifted it up. Get your feet as close as possible to where you will be placing the load, and try not to stick your chin forward as you put it down.

■ TOOLS

Are you using the right tools for the job? I know that it sounds obvious, but if you are working with tools that are not right for the job, it will have an effect on your body. You may notice this even if you only need to use them occasionally, but the impact is likely to be very significant if you are working with them every day. Most yards have many different types of forks and shovels lying around, but are you choosing the one that is most appropriate for your job?

Then there is the size of the tool that you have chosen relative to your size. Depending on the make, the length of the handle and the overall

weight can vary tremendously. Using something that is too heavy for you even without the added weight of wet straw is asking for trouble. And there is no point in following all the lifting advice to save your back if you are then using a tool with a handle that is too short. So when you are buying new tools, try to go to a larger store with a wide choice so that you can try out different tools, even if you don't actually end up purchasing them from there.

The next thing to check is whether your tool is broken. Even a small defect such as a loose screw can result in you having to work a lot harder and possibly straining your body. For the sake of a few extra minutes, it is worth either fixing the problem or finding a different tool.

Examples of this that I have seen are forks that rotate slightly as you load them, so that you have to twist in the opposite direction to stop the muck falling off. Or the broom where the head keeps dropping off if you sweep at the wrong angle, so you have to do a strange twisting action to keep it in place. I am sure that you could name plenty of quirky tools that you have put up with to the detriment of your body.

■ WATER CONTAINERS

How do you fill your water containers? I have seen so many people lifting or dragging them from the tap to the field or stall, and every time I have to stop myself from giving a lecture on how bad it is for their backs. Even if you meticulously follow every step of how to lift correctly, moving full water containers by yourself is a bad idea. Not only is water very heavy, but once the full container is moving the water starts to slop around, which makes the whole thing more unstable. There are several back-friendly alternatives that can be made practical so that they don't take up too much time.

The quickest solution is to ask for help. Two people carrying the water is a much safer technique, and you could help each other.

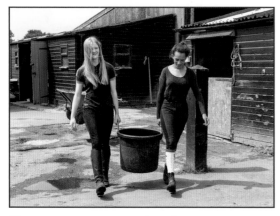

Carrying a water container the safe way.

The other simple way is to use smaller buckets to fill the large container. If the tap isn't too far from the container, then carrying a bucket in each hand doesn't normally place too much strain on your back, as long as you remember to pick them up correctly and not rush. For longer journeys using a trolley to transport the buckets is a safer way, but beware of potholes and muddy puddles.

If none of these suggestions are practical for your yard, then it would be very beneficial to look into an automatic drinker system for the stalls and field. Just think of how much pain and time you would save yourself.

■ MUCKING OUT

The key to mucking out without pain is to be willing to alter how you approach it. By making some slight changes to your routine, it is possible to get the job done in a way that is kinder to your body. So here are my top tips for mucking out:

1. **Check your tools:** Are you using the right type of fork for the bedding that your horse has? Are the tools the right size for you? Are all the tools in good working order?

2. **Wheelbarrows:** How many wheelbarrows on your yard have a flat tire, are cracked, or have a broken handle? Using a wheelbarrow that is broken immediately puts strain on your whole body, as you have to work so much harder to keep it upright and to wheel it in a straight line. Then you load it (or overload it) and it all goes wrong. So to protect your back and shoulders, only use a wheelbarrow that is in good working order and never put too much into it. When you are pushing a loaded wheelbarrow, try to keep your shoulders relaxed and look straight ahead. Lift the handles enough so that you do not have to bend your back to reach them. Use the power of your hips to push forward, not just your arms. If you feel that your back is tightening up, have a rest.

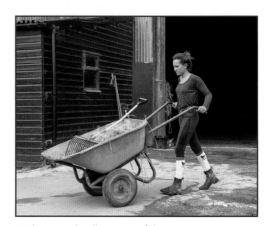

Pushing a wheelbarrow safely.

3. **Listen to your body:** As soon as you become aware that any muscles are starting to tighten up, you need to stop what you

are doing. But that does not necessarily mean stopping altogether. You could take a quick break to stretch the part of you that you are feeling, or swap to a different job. For example, stop forking up and do a bit of sweeping or empty the wheelbarrow. Basically, your body does not like repetitive movements, so if you continue to do the same thing while ignoring the warning signs, your body will gradually get tighter and tighter and then more and more painful until you are forced to stop. Then you are likely to have a flare up of existing problems or overstretch and injure yourself. If you can get your head around working in this way—following what your body is telling you instead of fighting it—life will become much less painful.

4. **Check your posture:** Do you look down most of the time when you are mucking out? As I said in chapter 6, your head is very heavy so looking down will drag your upper body forward, causing tension and pain in your upper back. Maintaining a good core position and glancing downward when you need to are the best way for any job.

5. **Lifting the soiled bedding:** Remember your lifting guidelines. The main thing to look out for here is never to stand with your back bent and then twist to one side to put the muck into the wheelbarrow. The photo in the section about poo picking shows how it should be done. Backs really can't cope with bending and twisting at the same time. Instead, once you have the loaded fork, straighten up and walk (or step around) to face the wheelbarrow before unloading the fork. Or you can position one foot toward the muck and the other toward the wheelbarrow. Then you just have to transfer your weight from one foot to the other.

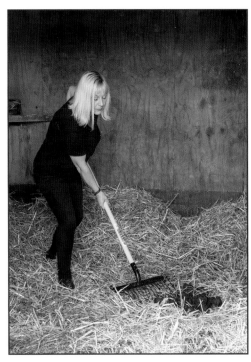

Mucking out safely.

6. **Look after your wrists:** Do you do the lift-and-flick maneuver? Again, it might seem more efficient at the time, but the repetitive way that it overloads your wrist joints will cause pain, inflammation, or even injury over time. Instead, use the power of your whole body when lifting and moving, so no one part has to take the strain.

7. **Sweeping:** This is yet another repetitive job that causes a lot of pain, even for people who do not have a back problem. Check the length of the handle, make sure there are no broken bits, and look at the head of the broom to ensure that it is up to the job. Sorry for repeating myself, but this is so important that I am going to:

Do not:
- look down
- bend your back
- hold your breath.

Do:

* look ahead
* stand with your feet pointing in the direction you are moving, with the opposite leg to the broom further forward
* transfer your weight from one leg to the other as you move forward and backward, instead of leading with your arms
* hold the broom with your hands high enough up to feel comfortable in your shoulders and back.

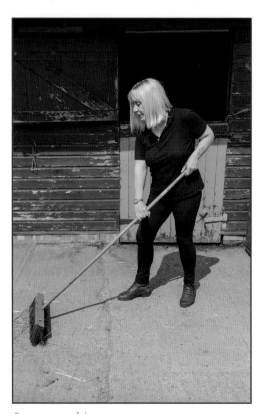

Sweeping safely.

Switch to a different task when you become aware of any tension building. Normally this will be felt between your shoulder blades or in your lower back, but the reason for it is pulling from the front of your body.

8. **The muck heap:** Forking up the muck heap is one of those jobs that can be very painful for many people, and it is a task that is often rushed. The best way to avoid the pain is, again, to take your time, take care of your back by avoiding bending and twisting at the same time, and rest when you need to.

■ POO PICKING

The term "poo picking" often conjures up an image of squelching across slippery fields in a pair of wellies (rain boots) while trying to push a wheelbarrow through water-logged muddy trenches. If you live in the UK this will probably be a familiar scene!

There are several things that you can do to reduce the impact of this job on your body, but unfortunately the biggest factor is the weather, which cannot be controlled. However, by planning ahead and being prepared, it is possible to poo-pick without increasing your pain.

Try to plan before starting so you don't have to carry a full container very far. Use a wheelbarrow if possible and, as I have already said, ensure that your tools are right for the job and for you.

Many people poo-pick without lifting their head or straightening their back up for most of the field. This may seem like the most efficient way of getting the job done, as you can always find the next pile of poo. However, how does it feel when you have finished? How many times have you been in the middle of a field with your hands on your back, trying to stand upright again?

So by simply standing up straight in between each poo, you will avoid getting stuck in that bent-over position and your back pain will not have a chance to build up in the same way. Look at the psoas muscle stretch in chapter 6 to see how to help your back pain while standing in a muddy field.

As I described in the how to lift section at the beginning of this chapter, it is important to change direction by moving your feet rather than twisting your back while you are carrying a forkful of poo. If you position your feet so that one is facing the poo and the other is facing the barrow, you will be able to transfer your weight from one foot to the other without twisting your back.

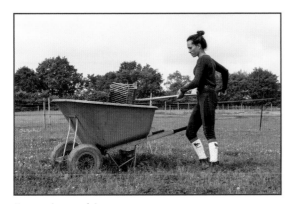

Poo picking safely.

■ HAY NETS

Giving a hay net to your horse may not sound like a heavy job, but it can cause pain and sometimes injury. Here are my top tips for getting hay nets to your horse without pain:

1. **Filling the net from a stack:** This can be tricky, depending on which part of the stack is open to take the hay from. Try facing in a direction where you don't have to twist to reach the hay. If you have to bend down to reach it, remember to bend your knees and stick your bottom out. You could also crouch

down or kneel to help your back. If possible, rest the net at the same level as the hay that you are pulling out to avoid repeatedly bending and straightening your back.

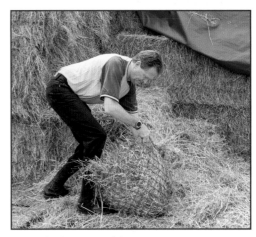

Filling the hay net safely.

2. **Carrying the hay nets:** If you have to take more than two at a time, by far the best way is to put them into a wheelbarrow so that you don't have to carry them. I know that nobody carefully holds a single net with both hands, close into the body—even I don't carry a hay net like that! But please don't sling several full nets over the same shoulder each time. The strain on your back, neck, and shoulders is huge, especially if you are repeating it many times. So, ideally, carry one net in each hand, making sure that they are not too heavy for you. You could also split the hay that your horse needs between two smaller nets to reduce the strain on your body.

3. **When you get to the stall:** Short cuts are not worth it. Open the stable door and tie the net at a height that suits you as well as your horse. Lifting hay over the top of a stable door and then leaning across to tie the net in place will tend to stir up any parts of your body that are problematic.

■ TRAILERS AND BOXES

Apologies for saying the same thing over and over again, but ... please do not lift the trailer to hitch it by yourself if you know that it is too heavy for you. Think about the lifting guidelines, positioning your feet correctly and controlling the lift.

The same advice should be applied to taking the ramp up and down and unhitching again. Particularly at the end of a hard day, it is too easy to forget how you are moving and lifting familiar things, and injuries can occur very quickly.

When you are maneuvering your horse in a confined space and you are focusing on keeping you both safe, try to also remember about your back position. So before you lean across to fix the head collar or lift the hay net into place, think about your foot position and try not to bend and twist at the same time.

■ GROOMING

As with mucking out, grooming is a task that often causes pain but that can be approached differently to be kinder to yourself.

Always be aware of what your body is telling you so that you can change the level and direction of the movement that you are doing. By mixing it up, you will get the same jobs done in the same time but without making your pain worse. (The same approach also works for gardening and housework.)

Here are my top grooming tips:

1. **Before you start:** Position your horse so that you have plenty of room to move around it. Having to work in a tight space makes it much more difficult to do things in a way that works with your body.

2. **Hoof picking:** Your posture is really important here. Either squat down or bend from your hips and knees and stick your bottom out. Keep breathing and soften your shoulders as you work.

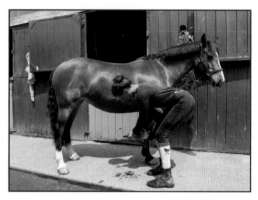

Hoof picking safely.

If the hoof is particularly tough to clear out, you may need to straighten up and take a break halfway through. Although this can be very frustrating, it is absolutely worth doing every time that you need to. Looking after your back at this stage can enable you to ride without pain later in the day. If you find that your fingers are cramping up, try using a differently shaped hoof pick, or turn it around so that you are using the pick in a different direction. Keeping your hands warm with gloves will make it easier too.

Now, here is the revolutionary bit—you don't have to do all four hooves one after the other! If you are struggling with your back or knees while hoof picking, change jobs after each foot. So you could brush the quarter of the horse that you are standing next to, then comb its tail before moving on to the next hoof. Try doing the psoas release from chapter 6 to stretch your back out between hooves.

3. **Brushing:** This is a good task to mix in with others when you are grooming, so that you vary the heights and angles of where you are working. Think about the position of your feet. As you change your reach, it is better to step around so your feet are facing the same direction as your body. That way you will avoid twisting and overreaching. Brushing feathers needs the same approach as hoof picking. As with hoof picks, there are many different types of brush that can be used for the same job, so finding one that suits your grip and reach is a good investment. Take your time; rushing will increase the tension all over your body.

4. **Plaiting:** How painful this job is depends on the relative heights of you and your horse. So use a step or grooming box to stand on to reach up or to kneel on to reach down if you need it. This way you will start in a good position that is less likely to cause shoulder and neck pain from straining to plait a large horse, or lower back pain from bending over for too long. Finger cramping will be worse in cold, wet weather, and plaiting with gloves is just awkward. So you may need to take frequent short breaks to stretch your fingers out before they reach the cramping stage. Try the finger stretches described in chapter 5. I have also found that putting little disposable heat packs in my pockets is helpful to defrost my hands when I need to.

■ TACK AND RUGS

1. Whether you store your tack in a dedicated room or shed, in your car, or at home, all riders inevitably spend a lot of time carrying armfuls of gear to and from their horse every day. The wheeled trolleys that are now available are the best solution to avoid having to carry heavy saddles. But you will still need to follow all the lifting guidelines from the beginning of this chapter when transferring the saddle from the trolley to your horse and back again. If you do not have a trolley, be prepared to do a couple of journeys rather than overloading yourself.

2. **Saddles:** One thing that I learnt early on was that it is easier to pick up your saddle the right way around than it is to have to try and turn it around as you put onto your horse! (I know it's obvious, but nobody told me when I first got my horse.) If you struggle to lift the saddle up onto your horse's back, have a sturdy grooming box handy to step up onto. Otherwise your back and shoulders will become tight and sore after a few times. But then you will need to bend down to catch the girth and do it up. So try to keep your hips and knees soft, sticking your bottom out as you reach forward. When you are holding the saddle, do not twist to transfer it; step around with your feet.

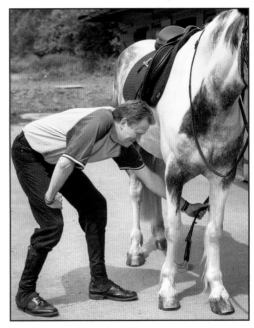

Reaching for the girth safely.

3. **Rugs:** Heavy rugs need to be carried in the same ways as anything else. Using the grooming-box step is also a good idea with rugs, and remember your posture when bending down to do the rug up.

4. **Bridles and head collars:** The most common cause of pain is having to bend down to reach your horse's head while fiddling with buckles and bits, and then suddenly having to follow it as it stretches its head up higher than you can reach. If you can train your horse to stand still with its head level, it will take a lot of strain off your body and make tacking up much quicker.

■ YOU AND YOUR HORSE

As I talked about in chapter 1, you and your horse will have an effect on each other, both physically and mentally, during all your interactions. It is well documented that horses are very sensitive to our emotions, and your tension will be picked up on as stress by your horse.

If you have anxieties around any aspects of dealing with your horse—for example, loading or catching from the field—this will probably make the situation worse. You can tell whether there is a physical effect by doing a quick body scan whenever you are in a stressful situation. Have your shoulders tensed up? Are you holding your breath? In this situation, asking a professional to step in with some advice might be the best way forward.

Tack

- Get your saddle fitting checked for you and your horse regularly, to take into account changes in both your bodies.

- If your stirrup lengths are uneven, get your pelvis checked.

- Keep an eye on the shape of the underside of your saddle—unevenness can be an indication of twisting in your or your horse's body.

Riding and leading at the same time

- Shoulders and back are the main areas of your body that will take the strain here.

- The problems come from one horse going more forward than the other, especially if it is without warning.

- So a strong core is essential in allowing the rest of your body to move with the pull without overstretching. Yoga and Pilates are great for developing your core in a safe way.

- You could also try some of the releases suggested in chapter 5 if any of the symptoms apply to you.

Strong horse pulling head down

- Riders who have to cope with this repeated movement often report pain and tightness in their back and shoulders.

- Apart from working with a trainer to reduce this behavior, your core strength is important again. If you are sitting correctly, you will be able to use the larger, stronger muscles in your core to maintain your balance when you are pulled. Then you will be less reliant on the smaller muscles in your back and shoulders, and won't need to have a tug-of-war with your horse.

Follow your body

- If you have any injuries, pain, or tension, then don't push yourself. Ride to your ability on the day, and get yourself treatment if you need it.
- Even if you don't have regular lessons, it is a good idea to get a friend to video you now and again. Then you can watch for asymmetries, rotations, and bad habits creeping in to your riding.
- Remember that if you are in pain or tight and compensating anywhere in your body, your horse will have to compensate too. Over time this will cause it to tighten up and possibly be in pain, and it will struggle to perform at its optimum level.
- If the horse you are riding is out of balance, it can also throw your body out.

Having to sit bucking, rearing, spooking, snatching horses

- This comes down to your core strength again, as the more secure your seat is, the more able you will be to withstand what your horse throws at you.
- If an incident has happened and you are aware of pain or tension anywhere in your body, it is a good idea to spend some time releasing those areas on the same day.
- For suggestions on how you can treat different parts of your body yourself, look in the index to find the relevant page in this book.

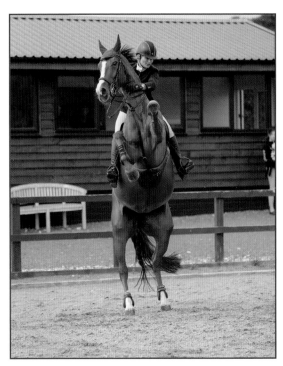

Photograph courtesy of Spencer Moret.

■ AT THE END OF THE DAY

Follow the simple steps in chapter 8 to help your body to recover from a hard day on the yard.

For tired legs: Lie on your back with your hips as close to a wall as possible and your legs up against the wall. Bring your legs slightly apart and roll your feet in to lengthen the outside of your feet and calves. You can then open your legs out along the wall to release your inner thighs. Remember, never stretch into pain, but find a tight point and wait there until it releases. This can be done on the floor or on a bed.

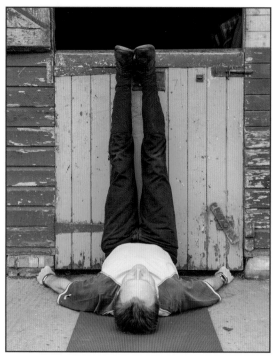

For tired legs.

Alternative release:

- Chapter 5: Fibromyalgia—constructive rest position

CHAPTER 8

Simple Steps

Please remember that the advice given in this chapter is general in nature and if you require individual advice, you should consult your own therapist.

■ DRINK ENOUGH WATER

Did you know ...

About sixty percent of your body is water, and a lot of that water is inside your cells. In fact, two-thirds of your cells' volume is made up of water. It is really important to stay well hydrated because every system in your body needs water to work properly.

What happens when you drink more water?

- Your joints are better lubricated, which allows them to move more freely and not stiffen up so easily. This can make a difference even if you already have wear and tear in a joint.
- Your digestion improves, as your body needs water to absorb the nutrients from food. Water also helps movement through your digestive tract, so it will help reduce constipation.
- All your cells can work more efficiently—they need water for all the chemical reactions that have to happen for your body to stay healthy.
- Your muscles are looser and more flexible when you move and exercise, so they can get stronger without being damaged.

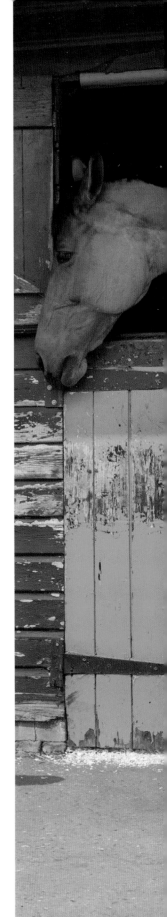

What if you get dehydrated?

There are some warning signs that should let you know that you are becoming dehydrated:

* Urine is a darker color than normal
* Low volume of urine
* Feeling very thirsty
* Reduced concentration
* Headache
* Dizziness
* Feeling tired or sleepy
* Dry mouth
* Dry skin.

Not drinking just because you don't have enough time or you are worried about not being able to get to a toilet is not a good idea. Some changes that happen in your body when you are dehydrated are:

* Your joints and muscles become tighter and less flexible, which can lead to them feeling stiff and sore. Any problems that you have can feel worse, simply because you need to drink more.
* You are at increased risk of getting a urinary tract infection (UTI).
* Cells can become damaged, which affects their ability to work properly. This can lead to your physical and mental performance suffering.
* Your body can't control your temperature, heart rate, or blood pressure properly, which can make you feel ill and can be very dangerous.

How to help yourself

Make sure that you drink enough:

* The European Food Safety Authority recommends that, each day, women should

drink about 1.6 liters (6.5 cups) and men should drink about 2.0 liters (8 cups) of fluid.[1]

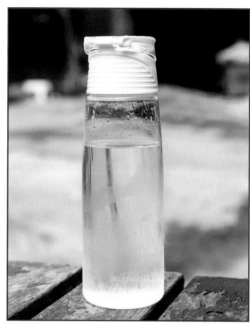

Take a water bottle to the yard.

* The amount that you need to drink at a particular time depends on your size, temperature, and activity levels.
* Any liquids that you drink count toward the total, but the recommended amounts are on top of any water that you might be getting from the food that you eat.
* All drinks provide water, but if you are drinking anything other than plain water, remember that your drink will also have other ingredients, which may include sugar and caffeine.
* Sipping your drinks slowly throughout the day is better than drinking a lot in one go.
* It is possible to drink too much water—if your urine is very pale and you are passing a lot of urine frequently, then you may be too hydrated.

Remember that healthy cells lead to a healthy body.

■ BREATHE PROPERLY

Strange as it sounds, there is a right and a wrong way of breathing. Many people breathe in the wrong way for their whole lives, and don't get any major problems. But if you already have an underlying condition or if you are in pain a lot of the time, the way that you breathe can have a big effect on the rest of your body.

If you have a history of breathing problems such as asthma, chronic obstructive pulmonary disease (COPD), pneumonia, or chest infections, you may already be aware of how difficult it is to take in a full breath of air when you are tight, coughing, or in pain.

Bruised and fractured ribs are extremely painful owing to the large number of nerve endings around your ribs, and because they are moved every time you breathe. The pain from these injuries tends to last for many weeks and your body will very quickly get used to trying to avoid movement in the injured area by bracing and taking shallower breaths.

If you have ever been winded in a fall, you will know exactly what it feels like to have the breath knocked out of you. As I discussed in chapter 3, the impact of the fall itself causes your body to tighten up and freeze, and that applies to your diaphragm and chest area too. If it is never released, you continue to breathe in a way that compensates for that tightness. How many times have you been winded?

What happens when you don't breathe properly?

If you are not breathing in as much oxygen as you need, and not breathing out enough carbon dioxide, your brain will make you breathe faster

until the levels are back to where they should be. This can happen when you are exercising, too cold, stressed, or in pain. But if you aren't breathing in the right way, it will occur more often. This can lead to you feeling very tired and short of breath, and tense and achy in your upper back and across your shoulders. It also makes pain, tension, or anxiety worse and harder to cope with.

If your diaphragm is tight and not working efficiently, you will end up overusing your accessory breathing muscles. These are muscles that are located around your chest and shoulders, and they shouldn't normally be used much in breathing. So when they have to take over they will tighten up and cause pain and tension in your upper back and chest.

So how should you breathe?

The diaphragm and the intercostal muscles between your ribs are the main muscles that should be working when you breathe in. Your diaphragm is a dome-shaped muscle that attaches all the way around the bottom of your ribs, in front of your spine and across the center of your body. Your esophagus (food pipe), aorta (large artery), and vena cava (large vein) pass through the muscle as it separates the top and bottom halves of your body.

When you contract your diaphragm it flattens, pulling your lungs down and pushing your abdominal contents out. This increases the volume of your lungs, decreasing the pressure and allowing air to be drawn in. That is why diaphragmatic breathing is sometimes called belly breathing.

Breathing out shouldn't take any effort at all; by relaxing your diaphragm and belly, the volume of

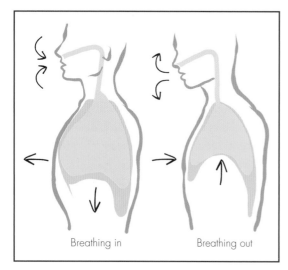

| Breathing in | Breathing out |

Diaphragmatic breathing.

your lungs will decrease, increasing the pressure and pushing the air back out. But remember to give yourself time to empty your lungs, so that they are not full of stale air when you try to take the next breath in. One of the problems when people hyperventilate is that they are trying so hard to take the next breath that they don't allow themselves to breathe out first.

You won't get it right all the time, as it takes practice to form the right habits and to retrain your muscles so you don't have to think about what you are doing. Just give yourself a few minutes every day to focus on it, and your breathing will improve. It is a good idea to practice diaphragmatic breathing in different positions and situations so that it is a more realistic scenario. For example, waiting at the lights in the car, standing to do the washing up, or lying in bed.

How to help yourself

As soon as you feel that you are breathing faster or using your shoulders more than your diaphragm for breathing in, focus on breathing properly until it settles down again.

An easy way to tell if you are doing diaphragmatic breathing is to gently place one hand on your belly, just below your ribs. As you take a breath in your hand should move up and out, sinking back down when you breathe out. Your shoulders shouldn't be moving much at all when you do this—if they do, just soften them and try again. But simply trying to push your belly out isn't going to work either, as your ribs should be swinging out at the same time. So focus on expanding your lungs, not your belly.

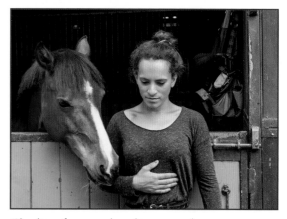

Checking if you are breathing properly.

If you are in pain whenever you move, the natural response is to tense up and hold your breath. This makes the pain worse, and you will probably end up feeling very tense and stressed. So if you expect it to hurt, breathe in before you start moving and slowly blow the breath out with your movement. You may need to do this in several stages to get to where you need to be, but that's OK. The main thing is focusing on breathing out and letting go of the muscles that don't need to be working. Don't take very deep breaths in each time though, or you may hyperventilate.

When you are riding

My daughter gets out of breath very quickly during her jumping lessons because she is concentrating so hard that she forgets to breathe. Concentration and stress are the main reasons why your breathing may be a problem while you are riding, and awareness is the best way to resolve it.

Try to get in the habit of checking how you are breathing while you are on horseback, riding at different paces. Does the speed change? Do you find it harder to use your diaphragm at certain times? Once you have identified where the problem is, then you can start to focus on your breathing at those times.

■ STRETCH

Have you ever watched a cat or dog stretch? They make it look like one of the most self-indulgent, luxurious, pleasurable activities in the world. And so it should be.

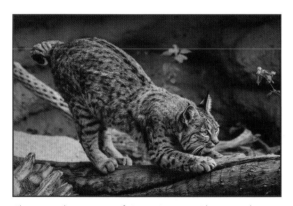

Photograph courtesy of @PeteMecozziPhotography via Twenty20.

Now think about when you woke up this morning. When you first began to move and your body began to stretch out, was that the moment that you got up, had a shower, sorted out the family, and started your day?

Imagine how it would feel to give your body just two minutes to be self-indulgent and to stretch

luxuriously before you got out of bed. So that as your muscles waken, they have the opportunity to open out and release the tension that has been building up overnight. Then, once you get out of bed, your body is prepared and better able to meet the demands put on it.

Your morning stretch and the stretches that follow a good yawn will change each time, depending on where in your body needs to open up. You don't need to know what to do, just trust your body and follow its need to stretch.

But there are times when you do need to think about stretching a specific muscle or area of your body—before and after exercise or if you have an injury or painful condition. This is when it is very important to do it correctly; otherwise the stretch will be ineffective or even cause damage.

Why do you feel tight?

When your body is loose, relaxed, and elastic, it can move and change with you. But it is very common to gradually feel tighter—this is often put down to getting older, but it isn't inevitable. As the pressure builds up in your muscles and they stiffen up, they gradually get thicker and shorter. This means that the blood flow isn't as good as it should be to help with healing, so you get more scarring, which makes the area even stiffer.

Some of the reasons for feeling tight are dehydration, poor posture, weakness in a different part of your body, not exercising properly, overusing muscles, and stress.

Remember that where you feel your symptoms is often different to where the cause of them is. Your tightness may be due to problems in another part of your body, and is your body's way of compensating and trying to protect itself. So there is no point in simply stretching the tight bit without also finding and treating the cause.

Stretching opens up the layers of your muscles, which helps the blood flow and takes the pressure off the nerves. So pain and inflammation can be prevented or improved.

How to help yourself

Give yourself time to stretch in the mornings and during the day. Whenever you notice that your muscles are becoming tight or restless, have a yawn and go with your body. Why not try it now?

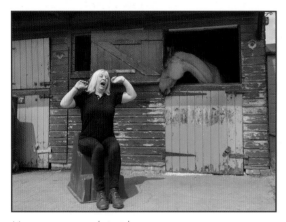

Have a yawn and stretch.

- Slowly open up to the point where you can feel the stretch but there is no pain.
- Hold there—never stretch into pain—your body's response to pain is to pull back, so it will make things tighter.
- Wait at that point until you feel the muscle release and get longer—if you don't wait for that change, you won't have stretched.
- Remember that each time you do a stretch, even to the same muscle, its requirements will be different. So one day it might release after thirty seconds and the next day it might take five minutes.

Chapters 6 and 7 show lots of different ways that you can stretch to help yourself to improve your posture and reduce symptoms. But they are just suggestions, and once you get used to feeling what your body needs, you don't necessarily need to stick to stretching in a certain position. As long as you follow the principles, you will do no harm to yourself and you will be able to identify and release tension before it has a chance to build up and cause more problems.

Yoga and Pilates classes are increasingly popular for people who want to have guidance on exercising and stretching safely. There are many different approaches within both disciplines, all of which have a place in the market but it can get confusing. I would recommend using a teacher who has training and experience in teaching people who have pain, as otherwise you may end up doing movements that are not good for you.

Finding a teacher and approach that suit you are very important factors, as you are more likely to be motivated and to want to attend the classes regularly. Small classes are generally a good idea, so that the teacher has a good view of how you are moving and is able to correct you quickly if needed. Whichever class you take, the rules of stretching still apply, and if your teacher is not willing to let you go at your own pace, please find someone else who is.

■ LISTEN TO YOUR BODY

Don't wait for pain—a lot of the time your body will start to tighten up a long time before the pain starts in response to activities. This is its way of trying to protect itself from overuse and injury, and if you respond to it straight away, it will relax again once the perceived danger has passed.

However, if you continue to do the same thing the danger signals will escalate and your body has to try harder and harder to get you to stop. If you ignore the tension it will start hurting, and if you ignore that too then expect a muscle spasm or cramp to stop you.

Animals are the masters of listening to their bodies and not just when it comes to stretching. Can you imagine your cat, dog, or horse staying in a position or continuing a movement that does not feel right or is painful? And there is absolutely no reason why we should, but we do! So next time you see your horse roll as soon as it is turned out, remember that it is following its body and releasing the tension that has built up.

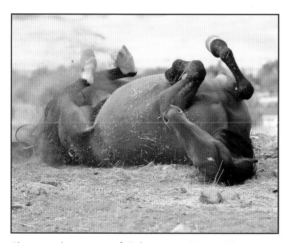

Photograph courtesy of @shaesy via Twenty20.

If you are willing to be flexible in how you move and work, your nervous system can relax and it will gradually become less irritable and allow you to get away with doing more. Planning activities so that you can change the height, angle, and timings to suit your body will give you that flexibility and save you a lot of suffering. Remember that just because you have always done something in a certain way, it doesn't have to stay that way.

"I'll just finish this ..."

How often do you think that and half an hour later find yourself in exactly the same position, doing the same thing? When you are doing jobs like mucking out, cleaning tack, or plaiting, it is very easy to get so absorbed in your task that it is difficult to listen to the signals that your body is sending you.

Whether or not you have a condition that causes pain, tightness, or fatigue, if you don't listen to your body, you will cause an increase in tension that over time will lead to symptoms. If you do have an underlying condition, it is even more important to listen to your body and pace yourself according to how you are feeling at that time on that day. It is normal for symptoms to vary from day to day, so you will find that your activity levels will vary accordingly.

How to help yourself

Take time to be aware of your body, particularly joints and muscles, during activities that you spend a lot of your day doing—can you feel areas tightening up after a certain length of time? This increased awareness of the changes that gradually occur during the day allows you to work with your body and to better manage or even prevent your symptoms from building up.

Myofascial release treatment can help your body to untangle so that it becomes the norm to feel loose and flexible, rather than tight. Then it is much easier to detect the early warning signs and to do something about them before they lead to a flare up of spasm, inflammation, and pain. There is more information about this treatment in chapter 9.

Asking for help isn't giving up. A lot of riders have been living with pain for a long time, and they just accept it. Changing the pattern of activities can be hard, but it is worth it in the long term.

Another common factor in symptom flare-ups is focusing on the amount of work or exercise that has to be done. So, rather than starting an activity by setting yourself targets of how long it is going to take or how many you are going to do, try doing it until you are aware that your body is starting to react. This takes practice, patience, and concentration to begin with, but it does get easier.

If a task feels overwhelming, try to break it down into stages that you know you are able to do. This even applies to something as simple as carrying a box across the yard. Plan where you can take a rest. Have a chair waiting for you when you have finished.

■ POSTURE

Even if you work with horses every day, your life away from the yard and horses will influence your riding posture. For those of you who do not ride for a living, outside factors play an even bigger role in how your body copes with riding and looking after your horse.

In the following list I have picked out just a few of the activities that can cause the postural problems that I see every day in my patients. If they apply to you, looking at the positions that you spend most of your time in will be helpful.

Computer work

Whether you work at a computer all day or just use it at home in the evenings, the way that your screen, keyboard, and chair are set up have a very real and ongoing effect on your body. People tend to get fixed in the same position after a while, particularly if they are concentrating hard or under pressure to get a piece of work done.

Your employer should assist you in getting the right equipment to be able to sit and work without pain, but if you are using your computer at home it is up to you.

Your seat should have good lumbar support (at the bottom of your back) and have adjustable height and tilt. If you need to reach to different areas regularly, having wheels and the ability to pivot is helpful.

Using a footrest, even for part of the day, can help to change your position and prevent your body from getting stuck in one place. If the height of the footrest can be changed too, that is even better.

Adjustable-height desks and workstations are becoming more popular and are ideal if you struggle to sit for a long time.

Check the levels of your screen, keyboard, and mouse. They should all be comfortable for you to use without straining—remember that if you share your desk with someone else, you need to recheck each time you sit down to work.

Laptops

Laptops should not be used on your lap!

As soon as you start to work from that position, your whole body is forced into flexion, putting stress and strain on your neck, back, and wrists, in particular. By placing your laptop on a table and preferably using all the same advice as for computer work, you will be much more comfortable and prevent many problems in the future.

Mobile phones and tablets

We are increasingly dependent on having access to technology wherever we are. It has even become normal to see riders (normally teenagers!) texting or messaging while on horseback. The main issue with this is the posture that your body is pulled into as soon as you look down and use both hands to type and hold the device.

If you're not sure what that is, try it now and focus on the changes in tension that you feel happening all over your body.

Some solutions are to limit the time that you spend focusing on your phone or tablet, place it on a table in front of you (ideally tilted up), or sit in a chair that supports your back and arms so that you can hold it up comfortably in front of you.

Holding phone between your ear and your shoulder

I know it is awkward having to do something with your hands and hold the phone at the same time, but please don't do this. It immediately causes tension to build up in both sides of your neck and into your shoulders. If you do it for long periods of time or on a regular basis, it will be very difficult to release that tightness yourself and it will be very likely to result in pain and headaches.

Using the speakerphone option on your phone, or investing in a headset if you spend a lot of time talking on the phone, is the best way of taking the strain off your neck and preventing a buildup of pain.

Driving

What sort of driver are you? If you are nervous, do your shoulders end up around your ears after a stressful journey? Do the other road users irritate you, making your own tension worse? What about when you are transporting horses?

I always ask my patients what makes their symptoms worse, and driving is one of the more common replies. Cars these days are much better for your body than they used to be, but only if you take advantage of them.

Some things to check and adjust in your car (apart from the mirror) are the steering-wheel height, seat height and position, lumbar support, and headrest position. Heated seats are also a great way of keeping your back relaxed when you are driving.

Walking dogs

Unless your dog is perfect at walking to heel at all times, you will probably have experienced that sudden pull up your arm and into your shoulder as he discovers a scent in the opposite direction that has to be investigated.

The first thing to try to do is soften your body and follow him—unless he is about to pull you off your feet. The natural reaction to a sudden change in pull or direction is to brace yourself, but that is when a lot of the damage can occur. By staying centered and feeling what direction he is heading for, it is much easier to predict movements and to stay with them. Then your body won't be as vulnerable to injury, as you will be more able to go with the pull.

Carrying shopping

Even if you only have to load and unload your shopping bags from the car, it can take a toll on your back. So planning ahead and taking your time can save you from future pain and injury. The main thing is to split your shopping into smaller, more manageably sized bags—that doesn't mean you can carry more bags at one time though! So be aware of your limits and be prepared to make more trips into the house with fewer bags, or ask for help.

Looking after babies and young children

People tend to hold babies in the same arm and sit toddlers on the same hip every time they are carrying them. When this is coupled with the bent-over posture that is normal when you are feeding a baby—either breast or bottle—you can imagine the strain that it puts on your whole spine. As a rule, flexing and twisting at the same time are your back's worst nightmare and it will complain if you keep doing it, especially while carrying a wriggling child.

Try to alternate the sides that you hold and carry, staying aware of how you are lifting the baby or toddler up from the floor, chair, or cot. If you already have back pain, try sitting in a chair and asking your toddler to climb up onto your lap. Then it is much easier to get your child into a good position and stand up.

If you are sitting to feed, pillows are the best way to support your arm while you support the baby. Sit well back into a comfortable chair with good lumbar positioning, and place the pillows under your arm and across your lap to lay the baby on. Remembering to breathe and softening your neck and shoulders will also help.

Staying in the same position all day

Whatever your job or hobbies, your body will react to the positions that you spend a lot of time in. My patients who teach young children, and spend most of the day bent over, all have back pain. Surgeons, dentists, and vets get pain and tension in their neck and across their shoulders from the position in which they stay when they are operating.

As with the computer work, the way to look after your body is to change position as soon as you become aware of the tension increasing, and before the pain sets in. Only you will know how to get round the problem, but it is very important that you do find a solution so that your pain doesn't stop you working—or riding.

Gardening

Again, planning is the best way to prevent problems when you are working in your garden. As with mucking out, having the right tools for the job that you are doing is an essential starting point. Then be prepared to chop and change what you are doing so that you do not repeat the same action at the same height and in the same direction for too long.

As soon as you become aware that any part of your body is starting to tighten up, that is the time to change what you are doing. Take a rest, get a drink, or have a stretch, or switch to a different activity. This should preferably be using different parts of your body at a different height. Then, once you have had enough of that action, you may be able to go back and finish the first task.

In this way, you will still achieve as much but in a way that is kinder to your body, so that you don't have to suffer the consequences the next day.

Listen to your body!

■ REFERENCE

1. European Food Safety Authority (EFSA) Panel on Dietetic Products, Nutrition, and Allergies. "Scientific Opinion on Dietary Reference Values for Water." *EFSA Journal* 8, no. 3 (2010). doi:10.2903/j.efsa.2010.1459.

CHAPTER 9

Myofascial Release

■ WHAT IS MYOFASCIAL RELEASE?

Myofascial release is a safe, gentle, hands-on treatment that works with your body to find and treat the cause of restrictions that lead to symptoms such as pain, tension, and inflammation.

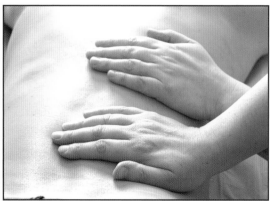

Photograph courtesy of Jamie Walker.

It was first developed around fifty years ago by American physiotherapist John F. Barnes, who defines it as an "innovative and highly effective whole body approach for the evaluation and treatment of pain and dysfunction."[1]

John Barnes suffered a very bad weight-lifting injury to his back when he was only seventeen years old, which left him in excruciating pain. Even when he had qualified as a physical therapist, and had tried many different treatments, he was in agony nearly all of the time. In his book, *Healing Ancient Wounds*, he describes himself as being in worse shape than most of the patients he was treating.

He ended up having surgery to remove a crushed disc and to fuse his spine, but although it reduced the intensity of the pain, he was still left with severe problems. It was at this time that he found a way to treat himself that lowered his pain levels and improved his mobility. By placing his hand on the skin and maintaining gentle pressure, he became aware of changes that spread beyond his hand and into other areas of his body.

He realized that he was changing his connective tissue, although at that time much less was understood about its structure and importance. By treating friends, family, and then his patients, John Barnes developed the techniques of Myofascial Release through trial and error. He was also treating horses in the same way with equally impressive results, and began to teach his methods to other therapists. Today, he has taught many thousands of therapists from around the world and his approach continues to teach, treat, and inspire many more.

Myofascial release is now used increasingly to treat competition, working, and general-purpose horses too. As with therapists who treat humans, more and more equine therapists are training in the technique and adding it to their skill set. Some are even treating both horse and rider, which is an ideal way to improve their balance as a team.

■ HOW DOES IT WORK?

As discussed in chapter 2, your fascial system connects every cell in your body via a continuous web of connective tissue, with the gloopy ground substance lying in between. The ground substance reacts to physical and emotional stress and becomes more solid, preventing your body from being able to adapt to things, and leading to symptoms and illness.

The ground substance is thixotropic, meaning that it becomes more fluid after 90 to 120 seconds of warmth and gentle, sustained pressure.[2] Once the pressure is removed from the connective tissue fibers, they are able to start to release, and gradually come back to their optimum position. This is why using a hot pack or having a warm

bath feels so relaxing, and can help to reduce pain and stiffness.

This property is similar to that found in Blu Tack (reusable adhesive putty); when it is cold and hasn't been used for a long time is it hard and ungiving. As you work it with your fingers, applying warmth and pressure, it gradually becomes more elastic and stretchy.

During treatment the warmth and pressure to start this thixotropic response comes from the therapist's hands. The therapist can use this reaction to feel where the restrictions are coming from and to gently follow and release them. As Myofascial Release treatment never forces the patient's body, it is very safe, and enables therapists to truly follow what their patients need, achieving long-term results. It also allows them to work very deeply without pain, so most patients find it a very relaxing experience.

By sinking down to the patient's barrier (as far as the tissue will give without forcing it), the therapist waits for the fascia to start to soften and let go. With training and experience, Myofascial Release therapists are able to follow the releases that occur and also to feel other areas of restriction in the body that are related.

In this way, we are able to feel our way through your tissues, releasing and then opening until the next restriction. As many symptoms begin in response to irritation from tightness in the fascia elsewhere in the body, it is usual for treatment to begin in a different part of the body to where the problem is felt.

Rather like unpicking a ball of string that is full of knots, it is important to release your body in the right order. The therapist is able to feel where the next knot along is in your body, and—just like the next knot in the ball of string—that may be on the other side of your body.

Some patients are very aware of the changes that occur during Myofascial Release treatment and are able to feel where in their body the therapist needs to work next. Others only feel the movement under the therapist's hands. Whether or not you can feel the subtle changes, they are still happening and are potentially altering your whole body via the fascial network.

■ WHAT DOES IT INVOLVE?

Assessment

The exact structure of the treatment will vary from therapist to therapist, but to give you an idea of what to expect if you decide to go for Myofascial Release treatment, I am going to describe what happens in my treatment center.

The first session always takes at least one hour, which includes assessment and treatment. We ask you to sign a consent form and you will be asked for your contact information and your full medical history. It can be helpful to bring a list of any medication you are taking. If you have a complex medical history you may choose to email it to us prior to your appointment, to save some time on the day.

Your past medical history is very relevant, as everything from how you were born onward has the potential to cause your fascial system to tighten up. So even relatively minor events and things that you may not have a memory of will be affecting your body today, and could be contributing to your current symptoms.

We will then assess your posture and look at any movements that are restricted by pain or stiffness. It is common for symptoms to occur in a different part of the body to where the problem originates, so treatment may not always be where you are experiencing pain. We will also check your pelvic alignment to see if that is having an effect on other parts of your body.

Myofascial release is a hands-on treatment that works best on skin, rather than through fabric. You may therefore be asked to take your clothes off down to your underwear, depending on the condition being treated. Some people prefer to bring shorts to change into—this is a personal preference. It is better to avoid using creams and lotions on your skin before treatment, as they can make your skin quite slippery when it warms up, and can make it harder for the therapist to be able to feel and follow your body as it changes.

Once the assessment is complete, we will discuss the treatment with you. The number of sessions required varies from patient to patient, even with the same symptoms, as the technique works with your body. As a general rule, the longer a symptom has been present, the longer it takes to resolve it. It may be possible to give you an idea of how many sessions you will require, but we cannot tell exactly.

Treatment

It is very important to communicate with us how you feel your treatment is progressing and what your expectations are. Myofascial release is not a "quick fix," but if you are able to complete the course of treatment that your body needs, it is often possible to get long-lasting results that

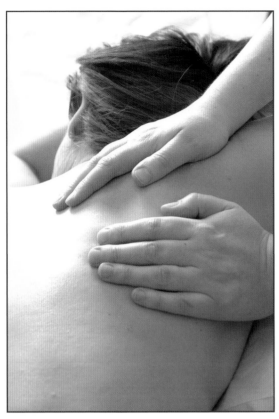

Photograph courtesy of Jamie Walker.

to know why or what event the emotion was specifically related to. In my experience, when emotions do come up during or after treatment, it is when you are ready to release them and it is never harmful.

Unwinding

Sometimes during your treatment you may experience movements that feel as though your therapist is initiating them. These are actually spontaneous movements known as unwinding. Animals and children do this naturally, they stretch and move without conscious thought as their body needs to.

Unwinding is a safe and effective way to release restrictions in the fascia by using the body's natural movements. As the restrictions are released your body begins to move, gradually self-correcting as the fascia returns to its normal state.

enable you to manage even chronic conditions yourself.

During your treatment, you are encouraged to tell us what you are feeling. This helps us to follow your body and also helps you to work with your body day to day. However it is important to tell your therapist immediately if the treatment becomes uncomfortable or painful, and you want him or her to stop.

As discussed in chapter 3, physical and emotional traumas are connected and are often held together in your tissues. So it is quite common for you to experience emotional releases during the treatment. These cannot be planned or predicted, and you do not need

What does unwinding feel like?

- It may feel as though you are moving in zero gravity.
- Your body feels lighter.
- You may think your therapist is moving you.
- You may get a tingling sensation.
- Your movements may feel jerky.
- Movements may become faster as the tissue releases.
- You may notice that your body goes into positions that you know you cannot do.

You may also feel that you want to cry, laugh, shout, or feel generally emotional. This is because as the fascia corrects itself, it may release the emotions that were present when the injury/trauma occurred.

Giving yourself permission to experience unwinding, rather than resisting, is extremely beneficial. Because the movement is coming from your body, it can never "go too far" and therefore will never strain or injure you.

Myofascial release is different from many other types of therapy in that the releases that start during your treatment continue for hours or even days after you leave. This is because the treatment changes restrictions and holding patterns deep within the connective tissue of the body.

Some people feel immediate benefits after their treatment, while others find that symptoms change over the next couple of days. Everybody will respond in their own way and you will start to learn how your body responds as you go through the course of treatment.

Following treatment, you may find that your symptoms feel as though they have become worse, rather than improving. This is nothing to be concerned about and is known as a healing crisis.

Your body is starting to heal itself, and this process commences with the elimination of toxins. When toxins are filtered into the bloodstream more quickly than they can be eliminated, it can make you feel as though your symptoms are worsening. You may also find that previous injuries or conditions feel that they are flaring up.

It is normal to feel energized, calm, relaxed, exhausted, moody, emotional, or anywhere in between. Try to tune in to your body and follow whatever is coming up—be gentle with yourself. To help alleviate the crisis, you should drink plenty of water to help your body flush out the toxins. You may also feel more tired than usual, so try to rest when you can.

A healing crisis is actually a positive sign: it shows that the treatment is having an effect. If you look after yourself it should pass quickly, usually in one to three days. Remember that healing is a process that will take time, and that it is normal to experience fluctuations in your symptoms.

Your therapist should be able to advise you on how you can help yourself at home in between appointments. This may include self-treatment techniques, stretches, or exercises—similar to those shown in this book.

■ WHERE CAN I GET TREATMENT?

There are growing numbers of therapists being trained in John Barnes's Myofascial Release in the US and the UK, and they will all have differing backgrounds and amounts of experience. However, if they are following the principles of this technique, you should be able to be confident that they will follow your body during the treatment, without forcing anything.

To find a therapist near you in the UK, I can recommend looking on the Myofascial Release UK website "Find a Practitioner" page: myofascialrelease.uk.

For therapists in the US, the best place to look is the directory on John Barnes's website: mfrtherapists.com.

My specialist Myofascial Release practice is called Holisticare. We are based on a working farm on the Hertfordshire/Essex border in England. All our therapists are trained in John Barnes's Myofascial Release, and our patients travel to us from all over the UK and Europe to receive our expert treatment. If you would like more information, please have a look at our website: www.holisticare.co.uk.

■ REFERENCES

1. J. Barnes. *Healing Ancient Wounds: The Renegade's Wisdom*. Paoli, PA: Rehabilitation Services. 2000.

2. H. Freundlich. "Some Recent Work on Gels." *Journal of Physical Chemistry* 41, no. 7 (1937): 901–10. doi:10.1021/j150385a001.

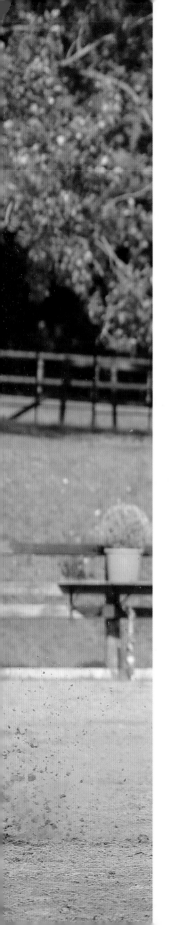

CHAPTER 10

Riders' Stories

For this chapter, eight of Holisticare's patients who are horse riders have told their stories in their own words. I asked the riders to talk about what caused their issues in the first place, how it affected their riding, their experience of treatment and the Myofascial Release approach, and finally what differences they have found it made to riding and caring for their horses.

I have included this in my book in the hope that their stories will inspire you to look for help for your own problems, and that they will give you hope for a future of riding without pain. Of course, the focus of their treatment is Myofascial Release, and I do think that is the best approach that I have come across. But there are many different techniques available and if you can find a therapist and treatment that suit you, please do keep trying to find the solution to your pain.

I have added therapy notes at the end of each story to explain some of the changes that these riders went through, and to relate them to what you have read in the rest of this book. I really hope that you find it helpful to read what other people have been through. If you have any questions about their stories or my comments, please do contact me through the Holisticare website, as I am always happy to talk about what we do and how it works.

■ JULIE'S STORY

I first met Nikki when she brought her horse to the yard I went to. We hit it off and rode out together. I gradually became aware that she was a Myofascial Release practitioner which I must say intrigued me more than a little.

Nikki organised a workshop at the yard over two evenings whereby riders could learn about how their own body with all the preceding "knocks and bangs" accumulated over a lifetime could be influencing the way they rode and have an effect on their horse's own balance.

It was the opening of a door; we first had to take it in turns to view each other from the front, back and sides, picking up mismatching shoulders, or turned out feet, hunched back or misaligned knees. Then Nikki and her colleague treated each of us for a few minutes. At the end they gave us exercises, incorporating a tennis ball to help to relieve and release the fascia.

Now my story begins I made an appointment with Ali. I'd been suffering with a lot of pain in my left thumb joint which I felt was being caused by some issues with RSI in my forearm. Ali worked her magic and the pain virtually disappeared, before I went I was wearing a brace on my wrist to try to alleviate the pain afterwards I didn't need to. After each treatment you are encouraged to drink lots of water as this hydrates the body and helps the fascia to keep releasing and freeing up problematic areas.

On another appointment Ali released my pelvis which was out of alignment and was causing me to sit lop sided on my horse, not to mention putting pressure on my hip joint which had also been giving me a lot of pain. A few years earlier I'd been to see an osteopath who had said I had one leg longer than the other which was causing me the pain in my hip. I was given an insert to wear in my shoe. This helped for a while but it was soon summer so I stopped with the insert because I wore sandals so that was that. After talking with Nikki and having treatment with Ali it become apparent to me that in fact my pelvis was the problem and not the fact that one leg was longer than the other.

I've since been back to Ali and had her help with other issues. Six years ago I underwent surgery to have a mastectomy and a tummy tuck to rebuild my breast. This left me with a scar which runs from hip to hip and also internal scarring which causes discomfort. Ali helped to relieve the pain and gave me exercises which can be done at home with a tennis ball.

I feel more balanced on my horse when I ride now, although I get stiff muscles in my back, which is caused by my psoas muscles being very tight. This is where the tennis ball comes into its own, by practising the exercises that I was shown helps to ease the tightness and release the muscles which in turn reduced the pain in my back.

I have lived with back pain on and off all my life, the light bulb moment came courtesy of Nikki and Ali, Myofascial Release treatment is fantastic and when explained makes perfect sense. I'm so happy that I met Nikki on that day over 18 months ago, and whenever I get aches and pains I don't feel any hesitation in booking my appointment. As well as relieving the pain it's a lovely hour of relaxation and special "me" time.

Notes from the author

Most of Julie's ongoing symptoms were connected to the strain put on various parts of her body by her rotated pelvic bones and the scar tissue. If her body had been balanced and flexible before the operation, she would have been much less likely to have problems from the scars and resulting tightness afterward.

Now that her pelvis has been balanced, it will be easier for her to feel when tension is starting to build up, and she will be able to do something about it before it causes other issues. Her riding will also benefit as she is no longer in pain the whole time and having to compensate for the painful movements and positions.

■ ALIX'S STORY

December 17th 2013 11.43am. I shall never forget this date. I was leading a horse to the field and the rubbish men were on the farm. I needed to pass through a narrow gap past them and I asked them to stop their truck – which they did briefly – but restarted it when I was only half way past. The horse spooked and crushed me against the wall. He pushed so hard I thought I was going to crack all my ribs. I was very lucky. I heard a big crack and thought xxx! There goes my collar bone but no I had a 3 part fracture to my right humerus right at the top of the bone, it was rotated and forced upwards. Shock is an interesting thing. The adrenaline kept me going to lead the horse with my broken arm 1.5 miles to the field. An emergency visit to Epsom specialist jockey fracture clinic then followed.

Thereafter started a four year recovery period. I say four years because the bones were healed after three months but the intensive rehab continued for six months, and I am still working on my arm to this day. I was told by the consultant in December 2013 I would only be able to lift my arm to right angles to my body. After four years I am almost able to do a full crab and can raise my arm above my head quite easily – it's not perfect – if you look hard you can see a defect but who cares – I have all the functionality that I need. I'm telling you this story as I think in rehab you need to believe in yourself. I had so many dark moments when I thought I would never be able to ride again. Thank god for pisco sour cocktails. You need to have faith in what you and your body can do. I have proved that I can do way, way more than what the NHS Physiotherapist and surgeon said I would be able to do – I am now back on horses, shovelling poo every day, lifting heavy things, running, yoga and my latest new year's resolution is to complete my crab goal.

Here is the journey I took: After eight weeks of sleeping bolt upright in bed, the fracture had reset itself into complete alignment without anything but strong painkillers and a simple sling. The consultant had forced me to do exercise from week two of the fracture – very gentle swinging rotations. They made me feel very sick. He thought he would need to operate but after four weeks the bones had set themselves perfectly all alone – all I had done was sleep bolt upright, done painful (!) gentle exercises and drank a ton of milk and good food. Then the real work started ... rather painful physio sessions and dedication and determination to do the exercises given. I found it very easy to say to myself well that's it, it's good enough when it was painful to do - I was lucky as I had my family pushing me to keep trying and saying "what if you tried this or that today". The thing that made the biggest difference was on month five post accident. I just couldn't raise my arm above my head. Here's where Myofascial Release came in. It was a stuck tightness that had developed from the outside of my right little finger twisting down my arm, into my armpit across the front of my body and down my left leg all the way to my ankle. And god that was tight. It was my body compensating and holding to protect the arm.

Between months five to twelve, regular Myofascial Release and continued dedication to the exercises released the last 30 degrees of arm movement. After that it was time to build muscle further to support the joint. It is so easy to get scared and stop moving but it's the worst thing I could have done. I would never have got to where I am now had it not been faith in myself and my team of Physiotherapy and Myofascial Release specialists getting me to push myself to the next step. I understood by the end that it's the little steps that count. If I reached too far for my body, it would shut down and I would spin back into a depression that I would never be able to do it. Small steps really helped me. Aim high in the long run, but take it in small digestible steps and don't rush.

I have learnt so very much about myself during this journey – it taught me to slow down for one and look at how lucky I have been. Even today, 5 years on, Nikki is helping me achieve my goal of full crab and being able to put my hands together behind my back in prayer position and slowly slowly the fascia is releasing to allow me to reach it. I hope my story will give you some conviction it is worth pushing on – just because one specialist says you can't, just don't take no for an answer – there will hopefully always be a way. I have since fallen several times on that same arm and it has held strong – a testament to the power and strength of a healthy fascial system.

Notes from the author

Alix's story is one of perseverance – both from her and from her therapists. Her shoulder injury was so bad that the doctors assumed that she would be left with severe restrictions, but they were focusing on the bony injury and not taking into account her amazing fascial system and determination.

Although the injury itself was to her upper arm, her whole body went through the trauma of that experience and the following months of pain. So if Alix had only ever had treatment on the painful area, her recovery is likely to have been much less successful. As she describes, the tightness that was limiting her shoulder movements was actually going from the little finger of her right hand, through her body, and across to her left ankle. If you imagine that line of tension in your own body you can start to understand how

important it is to have a "whole-body" approach to treating injuries.

■ SUSAN'S STORY

I have been having Myofascial Release treatment for the past year, alongside the fourth year of having regular weekly riding lessons of 2/3 hours.

It has been a joy and an amazing journey of connecting and healing my body, and seeing the dynamic results of how this benefits both myself, the riding and the relationship with the horse.

At the beginning of last year I had issues of a tight neck, stiffness across my shoulders travelling through to both of my arms. This directly affected how tightly I held onto the reins and was able to move with the direction of the horse. As this was freed up through the therapy, I had a lighter touch and was able to direct the horse more softly with less tension for both of us.

I have also had my pelvis realigned and the abdominal muscles, intestines and hip area worked on – so much tension has been able to be released. This has brought about such an improvement to me as a rider to be able to move more freely and feel the horse, as well as being more balanced and this in turn is kinder for the horse.

It's ongoing for me as the horse/pony shows up areas of imbalance and tightness in my body that affects my riding ability and I continue therapy.

Notes from the author

Susan had noticed that her pain and tightness were beginning to hold back her improvement in riding ability, and were also affecting how she was able to respond to the horse that she was riding. Tension may be held within your body for many different reasons, and you may not even be aware of what caused it or why you are still holding onto it. Luckily, you do not need to know the answer in order to let your tension go. As Susan experienced, your new freedom of movement and touch will directly benefit your riding and your relationship with your horse.

■ KYLE'S STORY

I first hurt my right foot/ankle about five years ago during a fall whilst skiing and I ended up with a rotational injury. Once home I took it steady for a while and did some stretching and rehab and was able to continue with my sports and activities as normal.

The second time I injured it was a year or two later riding my friends horse, Daisy. She managed to wedge my foot between herself and a gate post, even though I'd moved it forward in front of the saddle, and I suffered another rotational injury to the same foot.

Following on from that I had a couple of unplanned dismounts (she is a bit of a buckaroo) which resulted in me landing on my right side again, and then whilst on a canal boat trip I had one foot on the bank and one on the boat, and my right foot slipped on the wet. I didn't feel anything at the time but the next day it swelled up and was like a balloon for the rest of the week.

Now in hindsight I should have sought some treatment at that point, as the foot/ankle was getting aggravated easily with any slight bump or twist, but life was busy and I just soldiered on.

The straw that broke the camel's back (so to speak) was one Summer's evening when I was hacking on my current ride, Jamestar, when he did one of his best impressions of a rodeo horse (flybucks, the whole nine yards) and then set off across the field. I miraculously stayed on, but my right foot had gone forwards in the stirrup and as I attempted to pull him up it injured my right foot and ankle (again).

Stupidly I just soldiered on. It's just some bruising and soft tissue damage I said to myself. It'll be fine in a few weeks. I even went hunting a week or two down the line. A few weeks later it wasn't much better, so I had x-rays taken, saw the orthopaedic consultant a week later, and was told that it wasn't broken and that I had extensive soft-tissue damage that would take months to heal, and to moderate my activity levels in the meantime. So I did.

Three months down the line, having started to increase my activity levels and progress my rehab, it flared up again. It got more painful and very swollen. So I had more x-rays and an MRI scan, which showed that I had actually fractured the middle three metatarsals in my right foot. They were starting to knit together, but the bottom line was that because it had been missed when it was first x-rayed, I had even more soft-tissue and nerve damage as a result.

At that point I knew the time for some proper treatment was long overdue, and Nikki at Holisticare was my first port of call! I also included some Acupuncture in my treatment plan too.

Initially, as Nikki and her team began correcting all the compensations I had created, and realigned my joints, I went through a period where the foot pain was considerably worse, and

I could hardly walk for almost 2 months, let alone ride. A good indication of how I managed to mask the real extent of the injury as I carried on 'soldiering on' when I really should have sought treatment much earlier on!! I really should know better I told myself!

I kept going with my weekly treatment sessions, and after about ten weeks did an intensive week where I had one session a day for 6 days to really try and move things forward. By month three I was back to being able to walk relatively normally and was able to extend my walking duration bit by bit. By the end of month four I was able to be walking in the mountains for up to a couple of hours (albeit cautiously).

At the time of writing it is now five months since I started receiving treatment from Nikki and her team. I still have a way to go and now fully realise just how badly injured my lower leg was. That said I did start riding again about three weeks ago, and whilst uncomfortable at times on longer rides, I am able to hack out again in walk, trot and canter without any significant pain or issues.

The really good news is that I am very aware that I'm sitting much better in the saddle. I feel straighter in my back, equally weight in my seat, and feel much more balanced. I've also noticed that my thighs feel more open, thus allowing my horse to move more freely, and I feel very evenly weighted into both stirrups.

My lower leg and foot movement isn't quite back enough to do any really schooling work yet, but I strongly feel that when it is, my postural improvements will greatly benefit my riding and my horse's way of going.

So I'm really pleased with my progress. Furthermore, and probably most importantly,

out of all the therapies and treatments I have experience over the years, I can honestly say that I can't think of anything else that would have gotten me to where I am today in my healing.

The gentle nature of the Myofascial Release treatment really allowed the gradual breakthrough of the layers of tightness and damage, whereas something more invasive like deep tissue massage would have just made it flare up again.

I'm very grateful to Nikki and her team and would highly recommend them to anyone with an injury or ongoing physical issue that prevents or inhibits them from doing the activities they love, or even from simply living a normal life.

Notes from the author

Kyle's story really does show how important it is to seek help for injuries and to keep going back if things don't feel right. It also demonstrates what a remarkable ability our bodies have in compensating for injuries and allowing us to keep going, even through fractures.

But if you have had years of pushing through and coping with an injury, your whole body will have developed layers of tightness, which increase as time goes on. This tension eventually starts to mask the original problem, so a lot of what you feel is from the compensation. As Kyle's Myofascial Release treatment started to release this tension, the underlying injury, with its chronic inflammation and associated pain, was exposed. When this happens, it allows the therapist to treat the root of the problem and then real progress can be made.

■ MARSHA'S STORY

After 23 years of sitting at a desk, working like a maniac in London (I had given up riding), doing competitive yoga (no one told me all those years ago it wasn't meant to be pushing yourself to the limit!), I got a frozen shoulder and my body had slowly shut down and I became very scared to move because of the pain. I felt like a marionette and that if I made too much effort I would fall apart – it was better to just stay still. Various Physiotherapists told me I would never be able to ride again. Rock bottom as far as I was concerned.

A holiday in Morocco after a ten year break brought me back to riding horses on the beach. I went three times and the gentle rocking motion started to wake up my muscles and show me that it didn't have to be painful. Since that holiday I have never looked back. I got back into riding, found an amazing Pilates teacher, a brilliant Physiotherapist and an even more fantastic Myofascial Release specialist in the form of Nikki!

It has taken quite a number of years to get back to full physical functionality. Patience and many backward steps with my body falling apart quite regularly, but then ever so slowly over time, less regularly and then the pains and feeling turns into different pains and feelings and becoming duller. The most extraordinary part of my journey to health has been since discovering Myofascial Release through Nikki.

Each treatment is totally different and depends on what my body is prepared to present on the day. I know this sounds really weird but I have remembered accidents I have had through the years, which my body has literally moved through the motions of each accident – one time Nikki said I have a twirling, spinning feeling and I

immediately realised that it was a skating fall I had when I was six years old. Another time reminded me of a groin injury I had completely forgotten about when I was a teenager, then there were the obligatory umpteen riding tumbles and minor accidents around the yard – all that hoicking and lifting and slipping over the years. In time, we realised many of the problems were because of my neck and the various jerks it received through falls. Each trauma has presented itself in the treatment room when it was ready to be released.

I have been riding dressage competitively for a number of years now and I'm finding my treatments help resolve any alignment, balance, coordination and square-ness problems that I may have and it is literally making enormous differences to my horse's way of going and you can literally convert that into extra points in the ring. I am truly bowled over the difference Myofascial Release has made to my life. I feel freer, more "in my body" and confident. God knows where this amazing journey will take me next.

Notes from the author

Marsha has described a journey that many of our patients go through during the course of their Myofascial Release treatment. Over the years that the different traumas and injuries build up in your body, their effects become tangled up with one another. So, when you have treatment on one part of your body, which you may relate to a particular incident, it will often lead to a memory and feeling from a completely separate occasion.

These interrelated restrictions will, over time, lead to a creeping pull within your whole fascial system that puts a lot of strain on your body and causes symptoms to gradually build up. The Myofascial Release treatment enables your system to unwind and release the pressure on your nerve endings and cells, allowing your body to heal itself.

▣ JENNY'S STORY

I came across you first at WoodFest in September 2015. I had a stiff neck that I couldn't move very easily and in a ten minute taster, Sally released it and that was the beginning.

I bought myself my own horse in August 2009. It was a childhood dream but not without its challenges. My horse was spirited, nervous and had various body issues that needed to be addressed. And that's what I did: spent time working with various body workers and teachers to try and fix her. As I watched the people treating my horse, I would stand with one hip jutting out desperately trying to stand still and wonder whether this would fix her.

It's ironic really how much money we horse owners are willing to spend our beloved, gracious and so deserving, animals whilst standing badly, feeling uncomfortable and wanting to just get on and do it. Thankfully, I realised that I also needed some help and with a good team of a Pilates teacher (who is also a rider), a riding teacher (who is very much about softness and rhythm) and a lot of curiosity, a Myofascial Release practitioner. Oh and a good dose of patience.

My riding teacher wanted my leg further back in the saddle. My Pilates teacher laughed and said you can't just jam it there. I felt confused and a little frustrated. Why could they not all agree and then I could just do it. Once I started the Myofascial Release, physically things started

to resolve themselves. (I had previously seen a sports massage therapist – who always painfully released the tension, only for it to be tight again in two days.) I saw Sally who released my psoas and leveled my pelvis. Tightness was released slowly and gradually. I lengthened my stirrups by four holes when my hip flexors allowed. It took a while to regain my balance, but I have. My expectations changed for me and my horse. I realised making our bodies stronger would take time.

The biggest realisation for me as a rider is this. If I want my horse to go "nicely", to carry herself with balance and cadence, then I need to get out of her way. In order to do that, I need to engage my core, focus on me being soft and wait for her to trust that I was going to stay just as I was. My horse is 17 and I am 47. We have many years of "training" to undo and learn to trust the new ways.

That means, I should focus on me and look after my body in order to get the most out of her. We both deserve it. I feel very strongly about that. It's an ongoing process of noticing areas of discomfort or pain in me, and getting it released. I want my body to stay soft, so that I can ride until I'm 90 (at least).

It's more than that too. Sometimes my treatment focuses on some anxiety I am feeling and we all know just how sensitive horses are to all emotions. The gentle release and ongoing care and support from the myofascial team give me confidence that I am doing the right things for us both and that goes a long way to build my trust in me, so that my gorgeous horse can trust me.

In short, I recommend Myofascial Release to support you, the rider. It is entirely possible that your horse is just fine the way they are.

The thing I have really enjoyed about finding Holisticare and Myofascial Release treatments is taking the time to identify the areas of pain or discomfort in me. This has enabled me to focus more on myself as a rider, meaning I'm more balanced and more aware of how important it is to feel good. The more balanced I am, the better my horse is. I am also more accepting that she can or can't do something one day, maybe because of a pain issue, so that's really helpful.

I think taking the time to look after me – I am worth it, in order to improve our relationship is really powerful. And that really helps. Oh, I feel quite emotional. I've just come out of a session with Sally. Pain issues in my right hamstring. Tightness up and down it, and my calf is sore. But I've taken some positive steps to making it better, which feels great. I am worth it. I pretty much love everything about this place. Everyone always agrees that everything's right, it's all OK. Makes me feel like I matter and that's a really nice feeling.

Fundamentally when you ride a horse, we spend a lot of our time wondering why is she doing what she's doing but what I have learned with my horse, is that I need to be right myself and she will come right when I stop interfering. Focusing on me and making me better, more fluid, less sticky spots, enables me to give her more space and freedom to move more beautifully. She now trots like she's going to stop every second because the rush and the panic that she had before has gone. And now she trusts me now and I trust me and it's more of a partnership.

Coming here for a year and a half and had maybe 15/18 treatments. Sometimes I'm not sure if I'm worth it. But it feels like a way of rebalancing my whole body and to start everyday afresh. And I love it.

Glad I came across you at Woodfest in September 2015. I think your staff are amazing and I'm very grateful for the help you've given me and my Mum and various of my friends I've recommended to you. Thank you very much.

Notes from the author

Jenny has highlighted the importance of looking after yourself as much as your horse, and her story illustrates how closely connected you are with your horse. But symptoms are not only caused by physical restrictions; your emotions also have a big effect on your overall health and your relationship with your horse.

As Jenny found, Myofascial Release treatment enables you to release both physically and emotionally, which then helps your horse to stay calm and relaxed. This also means that any treatment that your horse receives is much more likely to be beneficial in the long term, as you are not constantly pulling it back out of balance.

■ CLARE'S STORY

I have had an intermittent 'bad back', for want of a better expression since the age of 17. I remember at school in sixth form having to sit whilst others stood to watch science demonstrations. If I didn't, within ten minutes, my back would hurt so much I couldn't concentrate. I navigated the university years pretty well, I played hockey for my college and represented the University for riding and modern pentathlon. In my final two years I was a Master of the University Drag Hunt.

Once I started working as a vet and then again after having children, I had a couple of bad episodes that lasted six to eight weeks. Then seven years later and four years ago I had been out on a trail hunt and got pulled by the horse constantly for a couple of hours. By the time I got off I couldn't stand upright properly, I was stuck bent forwards. So I laid down on the floor of the horse lorry and waited for it to pass, it didn't. I got home and gave myself a few days off and booked myself in to see a Physiotherapist. There was no improvement so I then added an Osteopath into the mix. Still no improvement. I then stopped riding because my back was so prone to suddenly ceasing up that it was a bit un-nerving on a flighty retrained racehorse.

After three months of various unsuccessful treatments I was really quite despondent. I was used to having a bad back that would last a couple of weeks and then improve, but if anything this was getting worse. It was around this time that a friend told me about Myofascial Release and she wondered if that might help me. I was so desperate that I was willing to try anything. I made a couple of appointments and was told that my pelvis was asymmetrical and if that was the case then all the other treatments were effectively treating the symptom and not the cause. The bottom line was that if the pelvis isn't straight then nothing else in the body will be either and the body will attempt to compensate for this and in so doing cause areas of tension and or muscle spasm. To my mind this was a logical explanation for what was happening to me, why my back problem had recurred and why it wouldn't get better.

I felt significant improvement after two treatments and after the fourth I was well enough to just book in to see the myofascial practitioner on a weekly basis. During the treatment itself I sometimes experienced a phenomenon called 'unwinding' which is explained elsewhere in the book and other times felt the tension go from a very tight area. Sometimes I never felt anything profound but the next day there would be a marked improvement. It was this that spurred me on to continue with the treatment. Within three weeks I was back riding again and have actually subsequently found that the horse's motion at walk is a really good way of loosening up the pelvis and lower back. In fact the treatment was so effective that I was able to cut down from monthly to every couple of months for 'maintenance'.

I have subsequently become much more aware of my core and how to engage it to protect my back and also riding using the core leads to a much more secure and effective seat. What I like about Myofascial Release is that it is all about getting to the bottom of the problem and not just treating the symptoms. This has meant, in my experience that once an improvement has been made it tends to last. I now go for myofascial treatment every two to three months as a maintenance treatment. I started practicing yoga which I believe has also really helped. My back has improved to the point where I am now riding every day, jumping, schooling, trail hunting for up to five hours and I am bringing on a youngster that has just been backed.

I was so blown away with the improvement Myofascial Release made to me and how I am now pain free that I have trained to do it in horses. My veterinary background means that I can assess if it is something that can be helped by Myofascial Release or if indeed the problem is needing veterinary treatment. Interestingly the principles are very similar and once the pelvic asymmetries are corrected in the horse they remain aligned and performance improves and tightness goes. In my opinion the rider and horse are inextricably linked. The asymmetries in one may lead to asymmetries in the other with a consequent reduction in overall performance of the pair. This is an exciting area to be researched. The gold standard has got to be for human and equine therapist to work together to help achieve the maximum potential from the pairing of horse and rider.

Notes from the author

Clare's history of years of pain, pushing through and continuing to ride, and then many failed attempts at fixing it is sadly a very familiar one to many horse riders. And, yet again, the changes came about once her pelvic alignment had been corrected, allowing the rest of her body to loosen up and strengthen in the right way.

Her insight into the importance of treating both horse and rider is fantastic. From her experience of being a patient and vet, she was able to feel the differences in herself and her horses. Now as an equine Myofascial Release therapist too, she is able to observe the relationship in her patients and their riders. I agree with her about the need for collaboration and further research into this area, so I hope that you will also be able to benefit from the resulting findings.

■ BETH'S STORY

I have suffered with a rotated hip and severe sciatic pain for many years. I had been going to a regular Physiotherapist and Osteopath weekly but still by the time I was home my hip was out of place.

Being a horse rider I was finding it increasingly painful to ride and my balance wasn't great. I have a very young horse I'm bringing on and because my hip was out he couldn't canter on

the correct leg as I wasn't able to give the correct aids with my seat. Because my hip was so far out that caused my left shoulder to be more forward than my right which then made my rein contact with my horse uneven … Again not helping with his straightness and the aids I'm giving him aren't clear.

A friend suggested Myofascial Release as it worked for her and I was recommended to go and see Nikki at Holisticare. I started having weekly sessions in November 2017.

The first session I had I felt very relaxed and was very different to the usual being pulled around that I had been having each week. The benefits weren't felt immediately however within a few hours the pain I had been experiencing got less and less.

On session three they performed the hip rotation to move my hip back in place, which again was very gentle. To my amazement by my following visit my hip was almost still in the correct place … we have progress!

I noticed with regards to my riding that straight away my horse was able to canter on the correct leg and my inner thighs felt less tight. My rein contact was a little better as well. I noticed that my seat bones felt level on the saddle and I wasn't tilting to one side anymore – for a little while this again made me feel unbalanced as my body was used to being wonky but after a few rides it felt brilliant.

I now visit Holisticare as and when I need a top up if I feel my body getting tight whilst riding. The improvement it has made is fantastic and that teamed with reformer Pilates has changed my riding as I have good core strength, balance and straightness.

Notes from the author

Beth discovered early on with her young horse the direct relationship between her body and his ability to learn the correct response to aids. Her rotated pelvis was also causing an imbalance in his movement, which in a growing horse could result in long-term problems.

The almost immediate improvement in his movement after her pelvis was corrected is a lovely example of how essential it is to treat yourself. The fact that she was no longer in pain when she was riding also meant that she was able to be more sensitive to his body as her pain was no longer taking over everything.

Bibliography

Davis, C. M. *Integrative Therapies in Rehabilitation*. Thorofare, NJ: Slack, 2017.

Duncan, R. *Myofascial Release*. Leeds, UK: Human Kinetics, 2014.

EDHS.info. "Understanding Ehlers-Danlos Syndrome Hypermobility-Type and Joint Hypermobility Syndrome." EDS-H & JHS. Last updated 2013, accessed 16 June 2018. https://www.edhs.info/what-is-eds-h.

Liptan G. *The FibroManual*. New York: Ballantine Books, 2016.

Mayberry, J. C., T. E. Pearson, K. J. Wiger, B. S. Diggs, and R. J. Mullins. "Equestrian Injury Prevention Efforts Need More Attention to Novice Riders." *Journal of Trauma* 62, no. 3 (2007): 735–39.

Pollack, G. H. *The Fourth Phase of Water*. Seattle, WA: Ebner and Sons, 2013.

Rashbaum, R. F. "Soft Tissue Trauma in Equestrian Participation." In *The Spine in Sports*, edited by S. H. Hochschuler, 180–91. Philadelphia, PA: Hanley and Belfus, 1990.

Robinson, C.-A. "The Psoas Muscle and its Role in Riding." Happy-Horse-Training. N.d., accessed 16 June 2018. http://www.happy-horse-training.com/psoas-muscle.html.

Sling the Mesh. "What Is the Campaign About?" WordPress. N.d., accessed 16 June 2018. https://slingthemesh.wordpress.com/.

Travell, J., D. Simons, and L. Simons. *Myofascial Pain and Dysfunction: The Trigger Point Manual*. 2nd ed. 2 vols. Baltimore, MD: Lippincott Williams and Williams, 1999.

Index